AGE IS JUST A NUMBER
DARREN MARTIN

Table of Contents

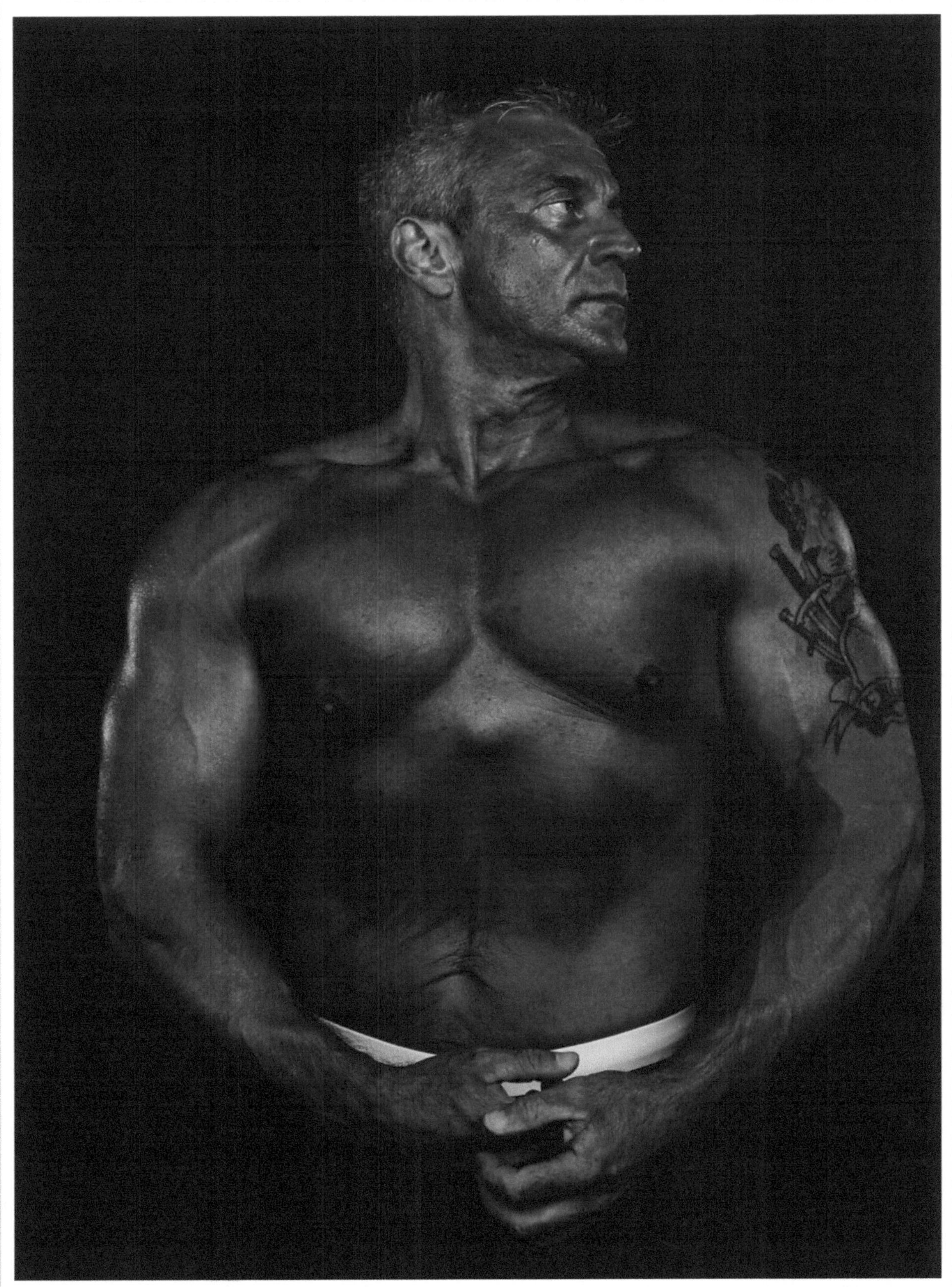

CHAPTER 1: INTRODUCTION

Where to begin…

I was always active, fit and healthy in my younger years: I played league football until I was 35, ran regularly and used the gym. I was quite lucky in the fact that I had a body type that didn't put on that much weight without being on a strict diet, however, like most people, that changed when I hit around the 35 year old mark. This milestone along with a football injury that left me unable to play anymore lead to something I never saw coming.

Over the next few years these factors alongside my hectic life of raising two teenage children and running my own construction company, my weight ballooned. I was eating more and what I was eating was unhealthy. Before I knew it, I was in the obese category and extremely unhealthy.

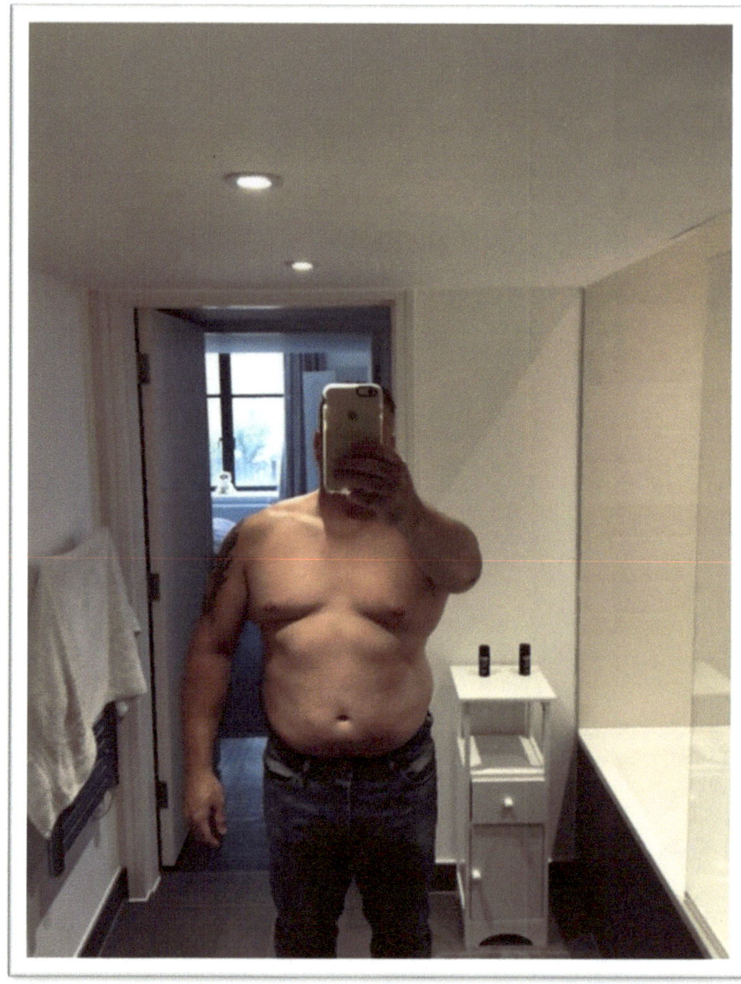

Most weekends were spent in front of the television watching shows or movies, and naturally this involved various unhealthy snacks and take away foods loaded with saturated fats and sugars, along with lord knows what these companies ram into our foods to make them taste good and (let's be honest) get us addicted to them. And that is exactly what we do become: addicted to these types of food and snacks – no different whatsoever to drugs, but more on this later.

This combined with the lack of exercise was only ever going lead to one outcome.

But for some strange reason you never see it coming. You start to look different, you certainly feel different but you don't see it, even when you look in the mirror, or worse: even when you're buying new clothes in the bigger size because the ones in your wardrobe are too tight. How on earth does our sub-conscious hide that one from us? Just one of life's mysteries I guess because we wouldn't do that to ourselves intentionally would we? But at some stage we do see it, we have to!

And it's at that moment you need to act.

Some call it a wakeup call, some an epiphany, "My eyes were finally opened," or even that "Life changing moment." Truth is, it doesn't matter what you call it, it's what you do with that moment and how you react to it that counts.

Mine was a strange one: a simple glance, or more a look of disgust (well that's how I saw it). I was sitting in a restaurant taking the usual large portion of something unhealthy, and a couple were sitting to the side of our table; I looked up and just caught the lady staring at my belly. Not much of a look, but enough for me to notice the look of disapproval on her face. It was then I realised my T-shirt had risen up over my belly leaving the stomach out and exposed, hanging over my trousers, it was pretty big anyway but sitting down it looked even worse.

Now some people may say, "So what? Who cares what a complete stranger thinks?" or "How rude to make a judgement like that!" and maybe I thought that at first, but then as quick as I did I also had my moment from the list of expressions listed above – my wake up call: "How did I get like this? How did I go from a pretty fit football player/gym goer to the 23 stone obese man sitting here? I need to change this, and quick." Unfortunately, some will just ignore this wakeup call (or whatever you want to call it), some will make excuses and continue down the path of obesity which only leads to one thing. . .

But since you are reading this book, I am guessing that like me, you didn't ignore that moment and you have started the journey to a fit, healthy and extended life.

Good, then let's get started.

Firstly, I would like to point out that this book is not aimed to give you all the answers in one go: because we are all different, with different body types, different types of problems and different levels of testosterone release and metabolism. I made the mistake, or many mistakes regarding this, trying to follow other peoples' routines and diets. But the truth is that what works for one person doesn't work for another. There were also the problems when starting on the journey with the 'advice' available always being tailored for the younger generation, say 20 to 35 year olds.

You've seen the types – they do 50 sit ups and have a six pack: that's not, nor ever is going to be us now. Also there were many people giving wrong advice or the advice they know you want to hear just to sell this protein or that energy drink. This quickly became one of my pet hates, and I began to see through the marketing and tricks and I could start to sense the difference between someone who wanted to give advice (I would like to point out that there are, if you look, plenty of good, helpful people as well) and provide help, and the ones that would tell you anything just to grab their commission from said product.

My other pet hate whilst I am on a bit of a rant is the training/exercise plans with the guy or girl saying STOP doing this it doesn't work or STOP doing that it is bad for you. Why? Why won't it work for me? Why is it bad for me? How do you know that doing crunches won't work for me or is bad for me? How do you know eggs in my diet won't help me lose weight?

Oh yes, of course, because you're selling your plan and you want to trick me into thinking everything else is bad just so I will stop and buy your plan. Absolute nonsense that really angers me.

There is no way that anyone, whatever their knowledge and experience, can generalise everyone in that way and put everyone in the same category. It's crazy, and worse, it's a con.

Yes, it's true that doing crunches can be bad for some people, but the same goes for any type of exercise or movement. This depends on how a person has treated their body in the past, and on any injury's they may have.

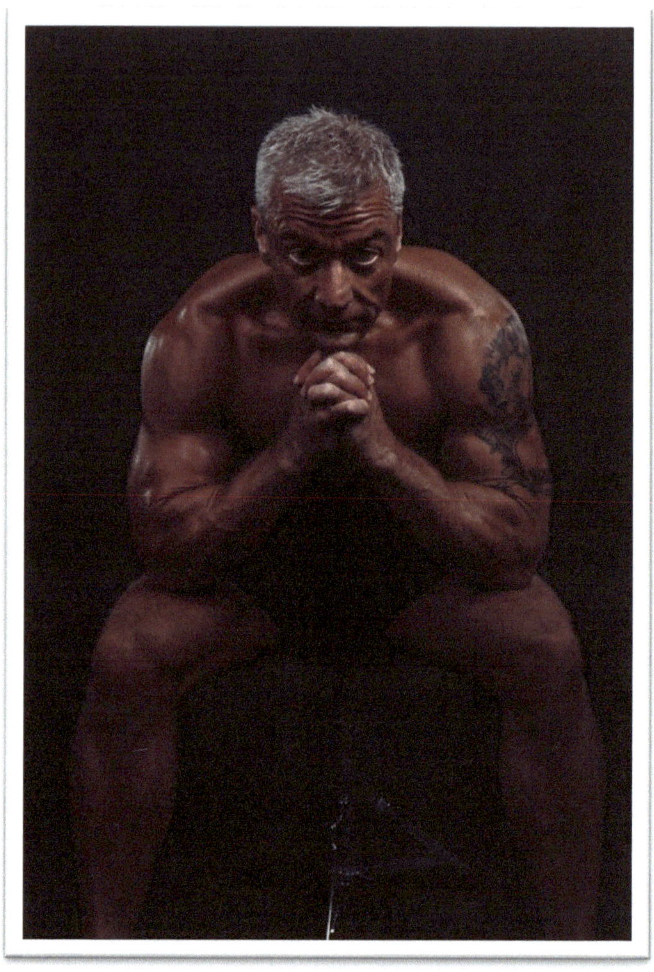

The fact is that without a personal consultation they have no way of knowing what affect a certain exercise could have on you, so the fact that they stand up in their YouTube channels and make statements of that degree is quite frankly a disgrace.

That same exercise you are being told not to do may work for you – you may get great risk-free results from doing it! It's the same with food, "Don't eat this or that, it doesn't help you lose weight, buy my diet plan, it will work for you!" Yeah, of course it will! Again, a disgraceful action.

As I said before I started my rant, everybody's body type and metabolism is different: some will eat certain foods and it will bloat them, or make their body hold water or slow their fat burn rate down, another person will eat the same thing and it could speed their metabolism up. There is no way to know without consultation from an expert, and to be honest, unlike the training part, this is even harder to detect without trial and error; and that's what I did, and that is what I want you to do, and by writing this book I will try and guide you through this minefield.

Unlike the exercise part where I took all different bits of advice and tweaked them to suit me, I did not listen to any advice on diet and food, and you shouldn't either. I am sure you are aware of fad diets: crash the weight off then it just comes back on. The makers of fad diets have no different agenda to the so called "experts" on the YouTube channels: they need you to fail and keep putting the weight back on to return for more advise and buy more of their plans.

There is one guy on YouTube that really gets my back up. He is so condescending and he doesn't even look good. There is one advert that comes on, and I was just in disbelief and outraged when I saw it. He comes into the kitchen with a big plate of lettuce in one hand and a full deep pan pizza in the other and says, "What are you having for lunch today?" He then throws the plate of lettuce on the counter and says, "Well, I am not having that!" He then goes into his speech of how he can change your body if you just follow his plan. Now here's the thing: he is still holding the deep pan pizza in the other hand. Forget the fact that no one is ever going to have just a plate of lettuce for lunch or even think that is the way to go, but what I did notice is he doesn't actually say he is having the pizza for lunch either, so why is it there? Because we are led to believe that he is having the pizza right? Otherwise why is he holding it? And there's the con. Of course he is not having a whole deep pan pizza for lunch, pizza is at the top of the list in the junk food chart for a reason, but he is trying to make you believe you can lose weight on his plan and eat what you want. This is complete nonsense and, in my opinion, disgusting behaviour. In this book I want to expose these people who take advantage of desperate people, like I was at that time, just to make money.

So, what's the answer? Well, it's a really simple one: work it out yourself.

If you think about it, the basics are pretty simple, you need to eat small portions of good quality food every 2 to 3 hours with a great mix of protein, clean carbs and vegetables. There is a diet section in this book which will go into more detail and tells you what I did and ate but what you will never hear from me in my training and diet advice is DON'T do this or that, that part is for you to decide.

So, with all that said, what is the purpose of this book? Well, the main purpose seeing as I have done this going towards my 50th year is to show that it can be done.

And although I am not saying you should do it exactly the way I did, you can take a lot from my diets and routines and shape them to suit you. In the end that's where I got to: I took a bit from this YouTube channel, a bit from this guy and a bit from that guy, tried them and thought: this works for me, I will implement this; or that didn't really work for me so forgot that one.

What I found out in the end is the diet and routine I will write about all worked for me, and once I had that formula, I literally felt and saw changes weekly, and that is a great feeling to have. Trust me when you feel it you will know exactly what I mean.

Another thing I recall was that most of this advice was not only for 20 to 35 year olds, it was also given by them (well, mainly 20 something's), so how was it ever going to work for me who was over 45? Hopefully as I have now turned 50 while writing this book a lot of it will work for you.

Now there may even be some of you who copy what's in this book to the letter, and if it works as well for you as it did me, that would be great, please let me know if you become one of them, as that would be another great feeling for me.

But don't worry about deferring from this book, that's exactly what you should be doing, until you have got your formula that's going to have you on the front cover of Men's Health (hopefully). I wish you all the luck in the world and stay strong, even when it's so hard you just want to give up, and trust me, those moments come quicker and harder than you first think when setting out on the journey, Remember, you will get past that point and you will find yourself even more determined and you will come out of that feeling and push on even harder.

Always set goals: maybe just a holiday, who doesn't want to look great on the beach right? Or a wedding where you can get back into your favourite suit, it can be literally anything, anything to keep your mind focused and not give in to the temptations when they arise.

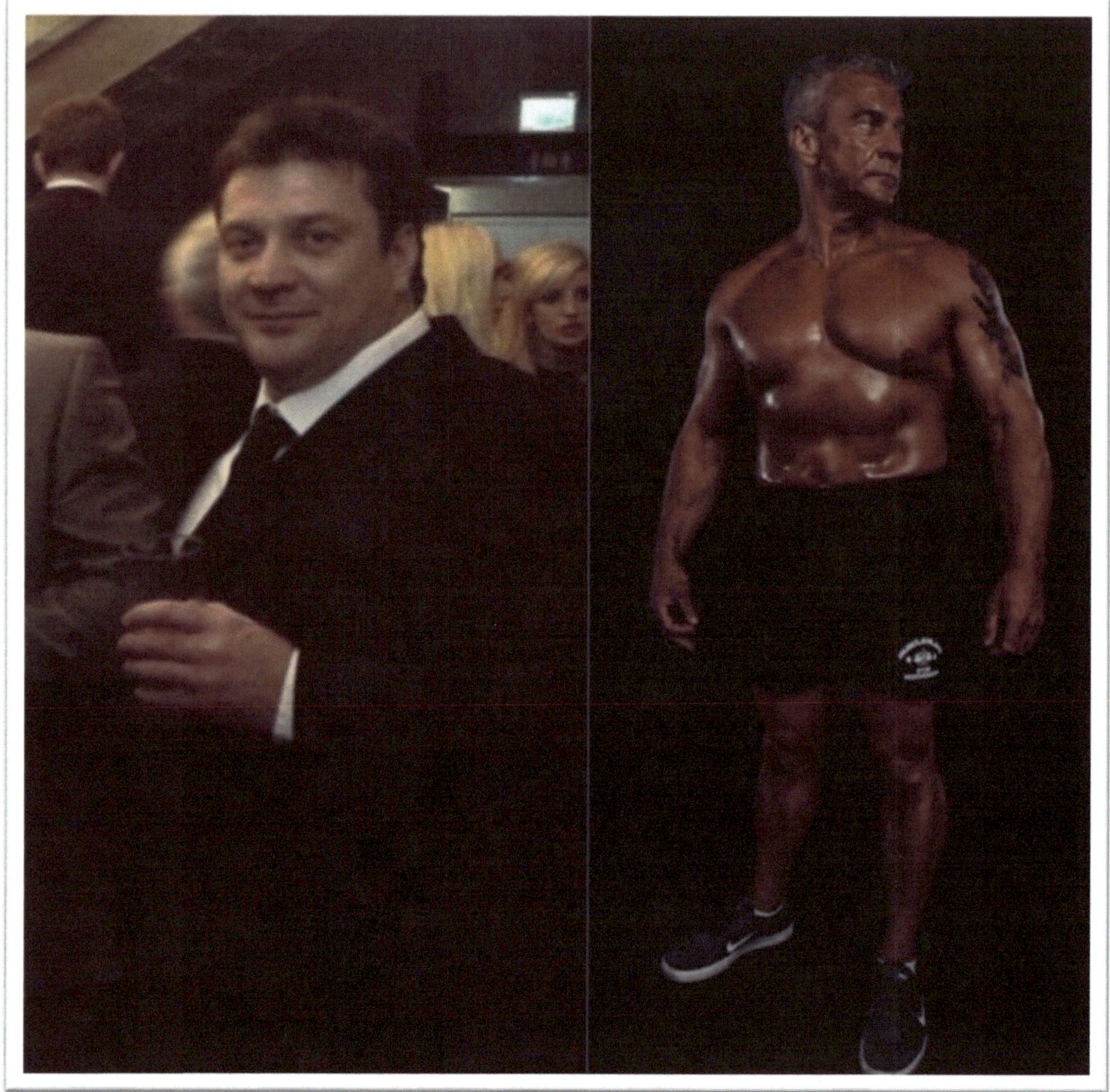

Mine was beach holidays to start with but then it turned into the ultimate target which was to release this book with a photo-shoot just after my 50th birthday. That worked a treat for me, it was good to have that set date.

Maybe you could enter a show, now the world of competing bodybuilding has developed allowing many more different body types to enter into various categories. Having a date where you will stand up in front of a crowd of people, well that's certainly going to keep you focused and on track no matter what comes your way. Like I said, I set my target to get to where I wanted to be as a photo-shoot on my 50th birthday, add the photos to complete this book and then a massive birthday bash to celebrate turning 50 with all my friends in Miami, also known as my happy place.

We had booked the hotel focusing on the type of pool party they held, that was going to be the big day, June 17th, 2020, a Miami pool party, until Covid 19 struck us all. In further chapters I will go into more depth of how this changed everything and how I, in spite of the ultimate curve ball being thrown at me, managed to keep on track with no Miami pool party to keep me on target, and worse: all gyms, swimming pools etc. closing and having to adapt to a whole new method of training and mind set.

Mind set is a big word when it comes to something like this, even without a global pandemic, sticking to your goals will always be hard. Hopefully by the time you are reading this book our lives will have pretty much gone back to normal. Everything that we took for granted and was then kept from us has now returned and we are all making the most of our lives, or what could be known I guess as our reset button as I heard a lot of people refer to. But this is a book in the fitness and health category, I will leave the philosophy talk around this global pandemic to someone much more qualified in that field.

The journey to a healthier and extended life is not easy at all, if it was, everyone would be walking around like a Hollywood star. It will take all of your determination, willpower and sheer grit to complete this, but I can't stress enough that if you make it to the end the feeling of accomplishment is off the chart. But to get there you will need to be strong and there will have to be a certain amount of sacrifice: when work colleagues ask you to join them for a drink or dinner after work; or you have a sudden visit from an out of town friend - but tonight is chest night, you have your prepped dinner in the fridge at home which you are supposed to eat 1 hour after training.

I want to make all these points as like I said at the beginning, I wanted to make this guide honest, and that is the fact of the matter: to achieve your goals you will need to say no, to the above and lots more, and that is the hard part – not the getting up early in the morning and doing the cardio, not the gym workout after work - it's the saying no to what before was the norm. Sticking to the diet – just because you think, "I have been good for a couple of weeks, this won't hurt," the truth is it will. You need to stick to the diet, training system, and most important of all, get the required amount of rest.

Well, hopefully I haven't talked you out of doing this, and hopefully my honesty hasn't been too daunting. No? Great, then let's do this, let's go on this great journey together!

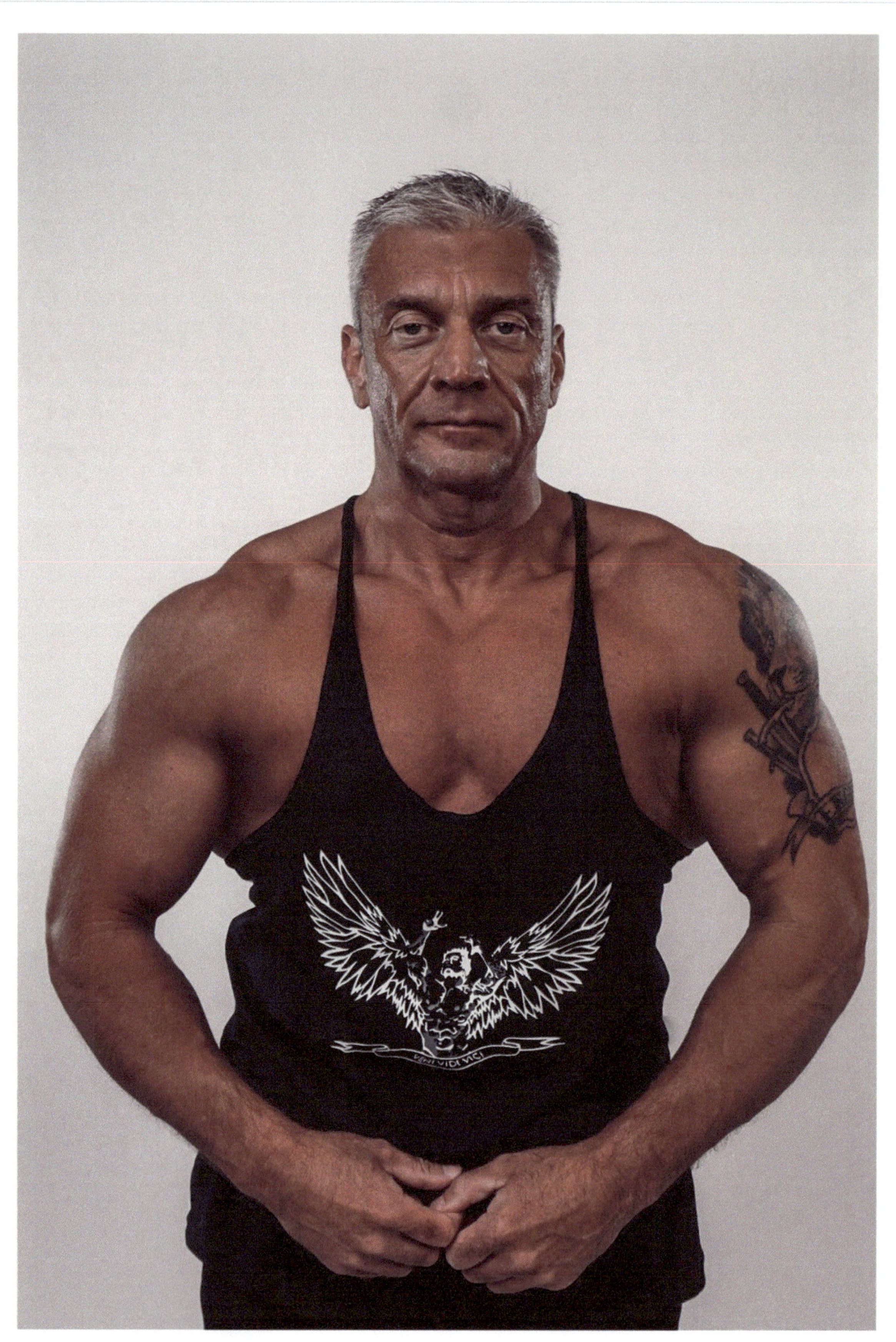
VENI VIDI VICI

CHAPTER 2: THE JOURNEY

All the ups and downs in what I aim to be the most honest account of my journey possible and what it felt like to finally reach the top of the mountain. I hope I can support you in your journey and meet you at the top, I will be waiting. Let's begin!

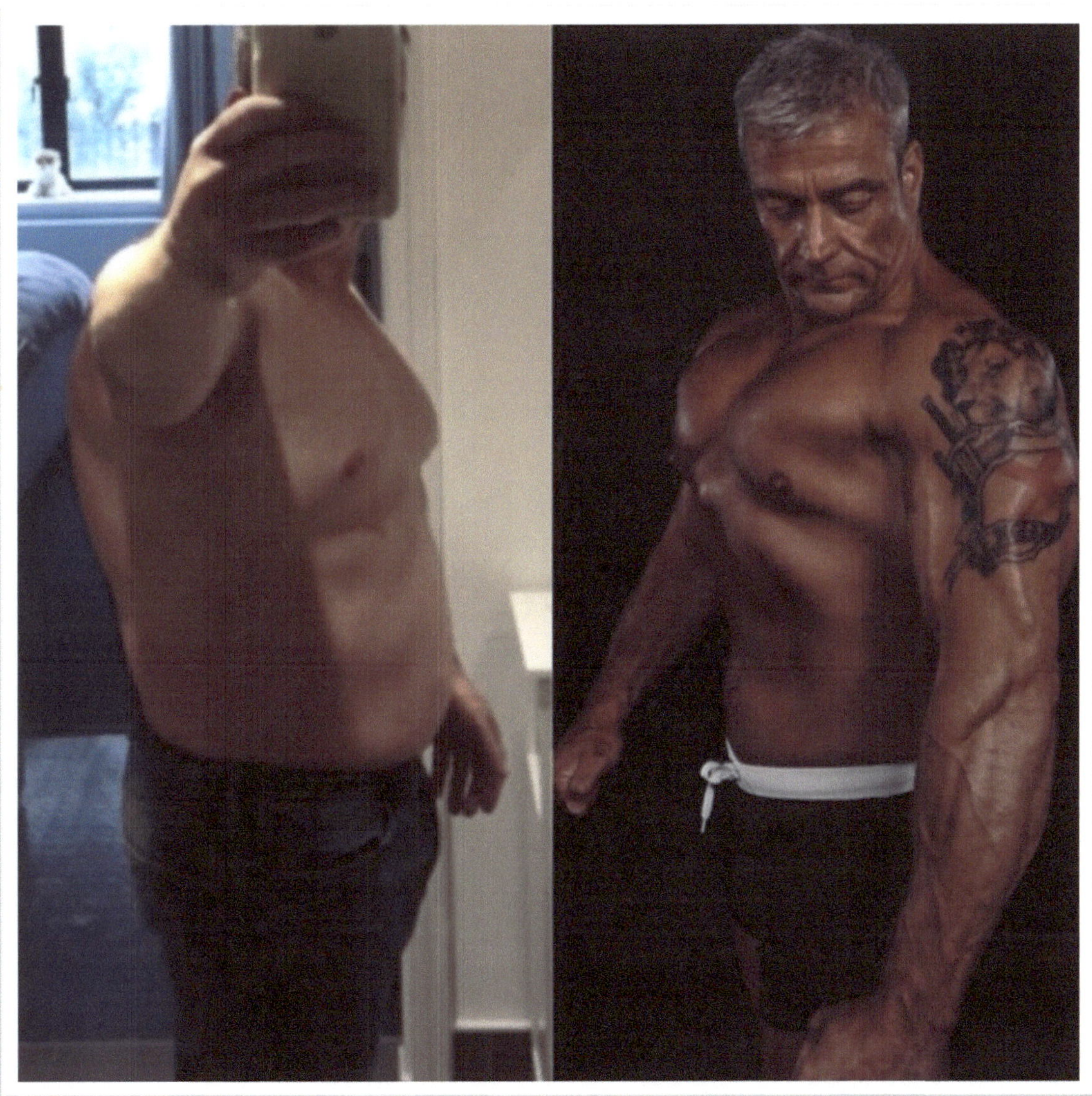

I think the biggest difference you will find between this book and others, or myself and other authors is I have done this process for real. I didn't put the weight on purposely (like some people have) to then straight away lose it to 'show how easy it is.'

Firstly, this is not easy, not by a long shot; and secondly there is a big difference between putting a load of weight on then dropping it straight away, and losing weight that has been on you for a long time which is much harder. I have also done it whilst working a very stressful and busy job – I am a construction project manager so I lead a very busy life and I understand fully how hard it is to maintain a fitness regime alongside sticking to a strict diet whilst working 10 hours a day and at weekends.

But this can be used as an advantage, it can put your mind into the right frame, you see, to get the results I have achieved you need to be disciplined and follow a schedule, again unlike other people giving advice on this subject (remember the plate of lettuce/pizza guy) I will be brutally honest in my writing in what this entails and takes.

I often found when busy with work my diet and training was spot on, because everything was done at the same time every day. I was able to perfect the perfect routine, that is the key word and you will hear it a lot within this guide.

Starting on this journey was just about getting back the fitness I had when I played football, but obviously the main goal was to lose the weight I had gained and to live a longer life. I have 3 grandchildren now which renewed a survival instinct in me, I wanted to be more of a father again than a grandfather, or the traditional type we think of when imagining these roles - play football with them, take them on holidays and be fully active with them, but mostly, live a hell of a lot more years to see them grow into adults than what my life expectancy was proposing in my current state, but, what transpired from this need was a whole different thing.

You hear it all the time, "The training bug." To be honest I wasn't really sure what that was until I got it, then a simple diet and training routine became a whole new beast. Your mind becomes set in a way where it is easy to turn down that invite to the pub after work, easy to say I need to do this but I will go to the gym first, and when you are there in that frame of mind, results are inevitable.

So, let's begin. . .

Getting up at 5am may seem like a crazy notion to some, I know that because plenty of people have told me so. But after lot of research I decided that fasted cardio first thing in the morning worked for me. What I learned quickly was that doing the same thing every morning didn't bear much fruit, and that's what I meant in the introduction about setting your routines through trial and error based on what I did, so you have your own perfect plan or you can follow mine, your body will let you know and guide you as long as you listen to it. And there lies a very important point that I can't stress enough: you need to listen to your body not only in the training schedule but also just as importantly where rest time is concerned.

I myself seem to be able to just go on and on. Some friends, training partners and especially my wife have often referred to me as a machine, this may be the case with you or it may not be. To get the required results you need the correct amount of rest as well as the correct amount of training, that part is crucial. Work through the pain barrier, push through your tiredness, and all the other phrases you hear around the gym are accurate, but only apply during workouts. If one day after work your body is screaming at you to rest, you need to rest. That is not something you want or need to push through. If in the morning when you wake your body screams that it needs a little more rest or a little more sleep then take it, your body does know best, you just need to make sure it's your body telling you and not your mind being a bit sneaky trying to trick you into just having a little more sleep. You will learn to know the difference trust me. Also, by listening to the advice your body gives you your workout in the next session will be that much better.

So, my morning cardio was a mixture of treadmill work, swimming or bike riding. You can add road running to that if it's not possible to get to the gym in the mornings to use the treadmill or pool.

I found these to be the easiest for the morning, If I didn't go to the gym I preferred the bike over road running as it's much easier on my knees and ankles which I did quite a bit of damage to in my football days (more about training for us older ones in the book later, as this is very important for our results). If you are the same, which let's face it, most men approaching 50 will have some injury's or restrictions, they need to be addressed when compiling your training routine.

As mentioned earlier, the Covid 19 pandemic put a stop to all the options mentioned above. Obviously, the morning cardio was the least activity hit as the bike ride and running was still available, in fact it was now something everyone was heavily encouraged to do. Remember the hour's exercise we were all given permission to do? But I could no longer do my uphill walking on the treadmill or the swim which was two activities I did have in my routine quite religiously.

So, the YouTube search began, and believe me it was quite the search. There are hours and hours of videos to sift through, even now that the gyms and pools are open I would still recommend to you to go through this process and look into the different types of exercise you can do. Firstly, because it makes your life easier as it can all be done in the comfort of your own home which also reduces the time you will spend on your morning cardio session; and secondly, unlike the diet advice, there are some great videos to follow. I actually learnt a lot from doing this and even now the gyms and pools are open I still do some of these videos, in fact as you will see in the training section later some mornings I just do some of the workouts I found, others I do a mix of the pool or treadmill along with the videos.

So, the first plus to being in lockdown was my morning cardio sessions have improved drastically.

Then it's breakfast time. I have always stuck to the traditional here: oats and eggs - simple to make and undoubtedly the best fuel for to replenish after your morning cardio and to set you up for the day. I did read a lot of different views around eggs, or more about egg yolks - good or not, and to be honest never really found a satisfactory answer. Some said skip them as they have too much fat, others said keep them because the fat content affecting your diet is a myth. So you know what I did? I did both. My breakfast contains 4 eggs: 2 I keep the yolk (these will disappear when you enter the phase 2 diet), and 2 I just have the egg white. Of course, now you can easily get hold of egg whites in a carton, most supermarkets sell them now, so rather than trying to find a supplement store to obtain them I just add them to my weekly shop which is great. No more trickery of separating the yolk from the egg with some expert chef manoeuvre, I lost count of the times that darn yolk popped into the bowl. I always poach the eggs, again, this is the best way and the easiest, a standard egg poacher with a 4-egg capacity is quite cheap and makes breakfast time so easy.

Along with 4 eggs I also had 75g of oats. There is quite a choice with oats, the only advice I would give is to stay away from the sachets, try and keep to the bags of natural oats and check there is no added salt or other additives. I always cook it the natural way in a pan, with 2 parts water, one part almond or coconut milk. I will go into more detail in the diet section but for now I do want to talk about measurements.

In the diet section I will be giving you the weights and measurements of all the food on my diet, but something that really frustrates me with some certain magazines who tell you what to eat weight wise, is this: I was 23 stone when I started this, I am now 14 stone, how could I possibly be eating the amount of food now I am 9 stone lighter and have completely different goals?

The same could be said for different body types: some people will burn more calories when training than others and have most people have different goals, that's why at the start of the diet section before we even discuss food you will need a macro calculator. These are available online, and you just need to put in your age, height, weight etc along with your goals and it will tell you the weights your food portions need to be to make sure you don't make all the mistakes I did when starting. This is so important, I can't stress enough that if you don't get this part right then no matter how much you train and how much work you put into this you will not achieve the results, it's that simple, it's that important. To put it in simple terms, put diesel in a high-performance petrol car and see what happens.

There is also a danger of over-eating even with good foods. I know, that sucks with a capital S right? How can that be? I change my diet and eat all the right foods and don't lose any weight or even worse I actually put it on?

As hard as that fact is, it is true and it is why many people that start dieting still get it wrong. You see, even if you eat say just chicken, fish, rice and vegetables, eating too much of this can still cause you to gain weight, which is why the following advice about counting and tracking calories and macros is so important.

Here you have 2 simple choices: old school or use the technology. For me I slowly converted from the former to the latter. The good news for you is I can now use my experience to lay out both options and with this part you can choose which one to do straight off the bat without the trial and error I have done.

So first, the old school option. As mentioned above there are plenty of calculators online to punch your details in to get you an exact guide but I will list out mine at the time of starting to give you an idea. Once you have your numbers I would suggest that even if you are doing it this way, still download an app on your phone which will calculate your macros as you consume them, and here's why: the calculator will give you the amount of calories you should be eating each day in order to lose the weight you set, whether that is 1 or 2lb a week. It will also tell you the percentages of protein, carbohydrates and fat which is far more important than the amount of calories - what you need to be aiming for is getting as close as possible to your daily intake of calories being made up of 40% protein, 40% carbohydrate and 20% fats. There is no point hitting your 2200 calorie target if there is 80% fat within that, and that is where the choice of foods comes in. To keep 2200 calories at 20% fat you can only have the good fats in your diet, this will be from your chicken and fish, for example. What the app will also do over time is educate you in what foods need to be in your diet and which ones shouldn't. Just for fun, whack that pizza into the app, when you see what comes out on the percentages and the nutrition value, trust me, like me, that will be the last pizza you eat! An example with me at one stage when I was 23 stone/146kg at the age of 45 my calories required came out at 3500, this means with the type of exercise I did which was set at high, 5 or 6 times a week, I needed to consume 3500 calories. So now you set your deficit depending on how quick you want to lose the weight, my advice is to set this realistically at first - you need time to adjust to this new lifestyle and get used to the different foods and exercise. If you try and set it too high to start you may burn out or just find you have had enough of this very quickly, depending on what you weigh and how much you want to lose of course, but I would just go for losing between half to one pound a week, and then if need be up it a little bit as you go and get more accustomed to this lifestyle.

For me that worked out around 500 calorie deficit a day which is a healthy and sustainable amount to get started with. Remember this is not a crash or fad diet, this is a change in lifestyle, so take your time, do it right and most importantly do it healthily.

The second option I mentioned earlier is to let technology do it for you which is what I progressed to and swear by today. I have the watch, scales and app which are all wirelessly linked. What this means is that whatever I do: steps, walk, bike ride, gym work etc. the watch tracks what calories I burn and sends it to the app which it turn tells me how many calories I can consume to keep to my goal which is now set at a maintenance level. I will tell you more about this in the last chapter, aptly called the maintenance chapter. This means I will never ever gain that weight again and will always look like the photos on the front cover, which was always my goal and is yours too.

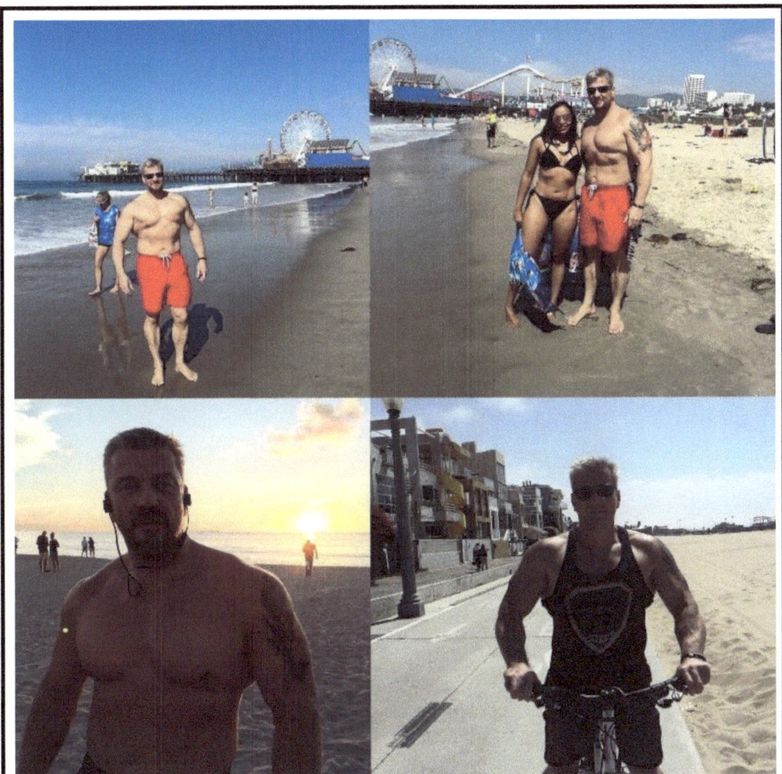

PROGRESS

As I started to lose the weight, I started to feel so much better within myself. The photos taken here were on trips to Miami and Los Angeles, well, where else would you want to go when you start looking good?

I would like to quickly point out something with scales though, like I said these are linked to the watch and app as well but I only use this part as an extra or little guide, please, please, please never fixate yourselves with scales and weight, it is only a guide to help you, the scales can lie and be misleading.

You may be holding some extra water when you weigh yourself, or you may be tired which affects it too, but more importantly it mainly depends on the body type you are trying to achieve. For example, if you look at my photos you will see of late I have concentrated on building muscle which weighs more than fat, so when I was losing fat and gaining muscle my weight went up even though I was shedding body fat.

Never get off the scales and say, "I haven't lost a thing this week, that's it I am giving up."

Remember the scales are not your friend, they will lie and cheat so look at them like that old boss you once had, he was there and needed but you were always going home that night and forgot all about him.

Be prepared to eat every 2 to 3 hours. The good news is there are only 3 meals that take any effort and time, so pretty much the norm in your lifestyle now (unless lunch is always at the local take away or sandwich bar, then it will be a big change): that's breakfast, lunch and dinner. The in-between ones are more like snacks, my mid-morning snack is always 2 rice cakes with natural peanut butter, make sure you are getting the natural peanut butter, the normal ones in the supermarket you may as well eat a bar of chocolate.

Speaking of chocolate, a little tip that I use is that I always keep a bar in the fridge, however, don't get too excited, it has to be dark natural chocolate and it also is just a tiny piece, one square if it comes that way - but it does carve any strong cravings should you get them and the right type of dark chocolate is good for you in very small portions. But like I said it is just one square, 1 bar will last me around 2 weeks to put that in perspective.

But back to the diet, lunch is pretty simple, I am quite boring in my food tastes which ironically makes dieting even easier. You are free to change but for me eating the same lunch every day has made it easy to prep which is the big thing. You see a lot of diets will have different foods every day, and there is nothing wrong with that, but, it becomes unmanageable if you have a busy life with work, family etc. To then add this amount of prep - its doomed to fail. The amount of people I have spoken to at work, in the gym etc. that were trying to diet, often resorted to nipping to the shop at lunchtime for one reason (or they say it's for one reason) - they didn't have time to prepare the lunch, or they ran out of something, that is the number one reason people fail - because they are trying to follow a plan that is just too time consuming and allows to many variables into the equation. So, an example, some diets will say you can have fish and veg one day, chicken and rice another etc. etc. Have you got time to make sure your fridge and cupboards are always stocked with that? No, no one does (excluding people that do this for a living), we have day jobs.

Now I know I take it to an extreme but it works: I have chicken, veg and grain every day, and it's all cooked in a steamer, and I can make 3 days' worth. So, compare my 45 minutes in the kitchen once every 3 days for the lunches to time spent prepping and making different lunches on certain other diet plans.

I buy the chicken in bulk direct from the source. I am lucky to live in the centre of London so a trip to the Smithfield's meat market at 3am is easy for me, but there are other ways to buy in bulk. A lot of suppliers deliver through their websites and there are some purely focused on fitness and bodybuilding foods. I buy my chicken once a month, spend an hour cutting it up, weighing it into bags and then in a freezer. Then every 3 days pop it in the steamer and I'm done. The outcome of this is you will never hear me say I need to go out and buy my lunch today, there is always a lunch in my fridge every morning to pop in my bag and go to work with.

My afternoon snack will be a whey protein shake or a small can of tuna in spring water with 2 diet crackers, they even do protein crackers now which is marvellous.

After work, its straight to the gym. I have never been one for going home first, then back out to the gym, especially in winter, that's a big no no for me.

So, what will the routines look like? The training guide ahead will show my routines that I have now put together in a rotating 4 week plan. I have spent a few years now trying different things, taking a bit from here and a bit from there and putting them together, trying different things and putting a lot of work into making what I believe is the perfect routine for losing fat and gaining lean muscle. Hopefully you will consider my before and after photos a good indication that I over the years achieved this and hopefully it will work as good for you to save you the trouble and frustration I went through.

There will also be a small section at the end on maintenance and what I plan to do to maintain my new look and healthy body, you need to understand that this is more of a lifestyle change than a diet.

I have split the 5 muscle groups into 1 group per session for 5 sessions a week, these are:

- Chest
- Shoulders
- Arms
- Legs
- Back

Again, this is my preference as it fits into my mind set and routine, but some do prefer to split them and do 2 parts in a session and do them twice a week, or some will do triceps in the same workout as chest and then do biceps within the back session which reduces your routine to 4 sessions of this type a week. Try all 3 options and see what feels best for you.

You will hear some people say you should mix it up and not do the same thing every week which is true, but for me the set routine is the key and what allows me to ensure I never miss a session. To get round this I will do the sessions as outlined in the training section on the same day every week but I mix up the actual session by changing rep numbers, doing different exercises and taking different positions to keep the body guessing on a 4 week rotation basis. I will outline all the different options in the training guide later.

You will be pleased to know my final main meal (yes, there is another meal after this but don't worry, it's the easiest of all) does have a bit more variety than breakfast or lunch. My reason for this is who doesn't pass a shop on the way home? Therefore there is a little more leniency as if you don't have it indoors then you can pick something up on the way home which allows for a little more choice, plus this way you can have what you fancy. Sometimes I go for the omelette, sometimes fish, You can see where I am going with this, it's not that I like to have to have the same thing every day, it's just that it works so well for me to stay on track.

There has been a lot of talk lately from various sectors that no carbs before bed is not quite as important than we have all been led to believe. I am still a little sceptical about that so with the exception of my prawn dish where I have a handful of rice, I still tend to keep my last meal carb free. I fill my plate with protein and salad but if you want to experiment and try a little carbs with the last meal try and see if that does work for you.

I think the diet community are still split 50/50 on this. The thinking was that your body can't burn the carbs when it's in rest mode - there is a lot of thought now that this isn't so true and your body will burn the carbs whether sleeping or working out. Like I said, this still doesn't sit right in my mind of thinking so my last carb intake is before my evening workout, after that it's all protein but feel free to experiment on this part to see what works for you best.

I do take a juice during the day but I stay clear of the fruit ones as the high content of sugar hamper the weight loss, instead I will use vegetables like carrot, kale or spinach, the carrot one does have half an apple in it, experiment with things like that using coconut water.

Sleep, I touched earlier on this and how important your rest was

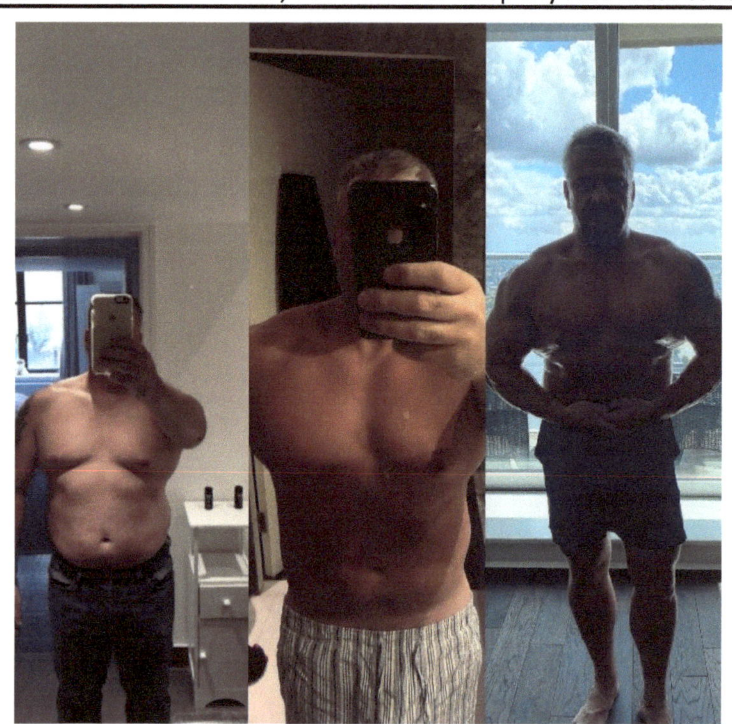

PROGRESS

Set of photos for start, middle and end (well, almost the end). This was about 2 months before the photo shoot. So glad I took regular photos as a record, this is easy to forget to do regularly but they are so important, mainly to remember your journey but also sometimes you will have moments when you wonder if all the sacrifice and hard work is even working - it's the mind playing tricks on you, having these photos are a quick way of looking back and saying rubbish, I am doing ok.

to achieve your goals, well sleep is a massive part of that, or more importantly how much you are getting. If you are the person who stays up till midnight, then this is not going to work. Any sleep expert will tell you that it takes a couple of hours to enter the deep sleep mode, so if you are going to bed at midnight, and it takes you 2 hours to enter your deep sleep mode (2am), and if like me you're getting up at 5 or 6am to do your cardio before work, you are running on just 3 or 4 hours of sleep. Forget the diet not working, I would deem you will struggle with your workday as well.

My routine has me hitting the sack somewhere between 9pm and 10pm, have my cup of red bush tea with a little reading then its lights out for 10pm. That way I am getting my 7 hours of rest with 5 hours of my deep sleep. This is back to what I keep referring to of habit - this has become my routine so just comes naturally which again is the key to all this: meals, cardio, gym work, sleep, it's all in a routine that allows you to arrive at a place where you feel straight away something is out when you miss a cardio session, miss a meal, go to bed late, it all registers straight away, like a warning sound in your head. Get to that point and you are now on your way to a better-looking body, a healthier lifestyle and most importantly, a longer life.

Curveballs. I touched on this earlier in the introduction, I also touched on the biggest one that anyone on a diet or training programme could face this year, or any year for that matter: Covid 19. Two months before my final milestone, the goal I had put all this hard work into, my 50th Birthday was fast approaching. This book had started to take shape along with my body, invites had gone out to all my friends for the Miami pool birthday party, WhatsApp group all set up, because we all know how important that is for a successful event.

I had just started to enter into phase 2, diet and my routines were perfect, then bang, we were in a pandemic.

Gyms closed, people panic buying so food types were running out – I remember going to the Smithfield meat market the week before lockdown was implemented, they had run out of chicken, imagine that, no chicken at all in the largest meat market in London. I couldn't believe it, and I guess it was the first thing that made me stop and think, "This is going to be a period in our lives like nothing we had seen before." And it turned out to be just that, it became apparent very quickly that we would not have access to gyms or pools or anything that resembled the way we have all become accustomed to training now. What was also apparent was there was not going to be any sort of 50th birthday party let alone a Miami pool party.

There was a moment when I just sat there head in hands and thought, "How do I continue with this? Do I just give in? All the goals are gone - no photo shoot, no 50th party and no facilities". That thought didn't last long. In the light of things my problems were so trivial compared to what people were going through: losing loved ones, losing their jobs and businesses.

Yes, my consultancy business did suffer from this but I managed to keep working as a consultant for 3 days a week which paid my bills, and ironically gave me more time to concentrate on finishing my goal – I could now do full 1.5 hour cardio workouts every morning as even the 3 days I did work, it was from home. All I had to do was change my way of thinking, change my workouts, do lots of researching of YouTube videos on home workouts. Resistance band training suddenly became the most watched videos on YouTube, which was a welcome relief from cat videos I guess.

Some home shopping for gym mats and bands and suddenly I was back on track. The panic buying thankfully went as quick as it came and people realised, they didn't need to rush out purchasing everything in sight (I am still refraining myself from mentioning toilet rolls). Everything I needed for the diet was all available again and it all worked out ok.

If anything, I think it helped me achieve the condition I am in the final photos, and here's why: sometimes in the gym environment it is easy to get caught up in lifting heavy. There are some big guys in the gym lifting big weights and, well, we are guys right, it's a macho thing, I am not picking up the 25kg when he has got the 50kg dumbbell! But now suddenly I was in a position when lifting heavy was no longer an option, cardio was king of these new workouts.

I did try and replicate my main body part lifts and exercises, but it was now with bands not weights so it was never going to be the same. It had to be much higher reps and less breaks. What it has allowed me to do is the workout I have provided in this book will work even better because hopefully by the time you read this book everything will be back to normal and you will have the full range of facilities available to you, I can now advise in this book and pass on what I learnt to obtain this body with my years of experience of gym work along with what this period of time in lockdown taught me. When the gym did open I was the first one back, but with a different view of what I thought was the right thing to do and it worked a treat – I actually printed out the pages of this book with the training section and went to work with it perfecting it even more.

Also what I did, and you should try this this even if you change some of the routines: I took the pages in and noted all the perfect weights by each exercise that either worked for the heavy sets or worked perfectly when doing the lighter sets for the full 45 seconds. That way the next time I did that exercise I would start straight off with the correct weight. It also ensures you are tracking your progress perfectly.

So that was an extreme curve ball and hopefully not one any of us have to combat ever again, but without Covid 19 I would still have had a section in this book about curveballs, so I will touch on ones that will come your way and the way to deal with them.

The biggest thing is when they do come not to beat yourself up about them. Quickly make a note in your mind of it and move on. The problem is we have a tendency to beat ourselves up about it because our mind tells us to. It tells us we need to be hard on ourselves as this will stop us doing it again, maybe something that resonates itself from our upbringing. The reality is the opposite: when we let ourselves feel too bad about our mistakes it leads to negative thoughts which then leads us to make the mistake again and even bigger. The idea is to spin it into a positive: I will work harder next workout, I will learn from this, look at why it happened, what were the circumstances that lead you there, once you have a plan to rectify eating that fast food meal by making a plan to work it off in the next workout and a plan to not put yourself in the situation that lead you there you have a positive thought about it which allows you to move on without forgetting the mistake, but most importantly move on without shutting off.

An example of this would be, imagine its Friday, you are just finishing work and on your way to the gym, but the work colleagues are all going out for a drink. Now I have been in this situation and I have been training a long time, and these people know that. Maybe that's the challenge for some people, maybe intentionally or unintentionally they are thinking, "Let's get this guy to break his routine, let's get him out in a pub Friday night instead of the gym," I don't know, maybe, but the thing is they do ask and sometimes quite persistently.

Now if you have just started your journey they won't know, or more like they won't take you seriously when you say, "I can't come with you I need to go to the gym." Maybe it's quite the norm you do go, but you are changing your life now, so how do you say no? This is where you will grow a little arsenal of your own little tricks, your response could include, "Yeah sure, I will catch you up, just need to send this email or finish this report," or, "Ok, I will come but I am just going to have a juice or mineral water then go to the gym after." They will obviously object to this and spill the line, "Have a proper drink," but this is where you need your strength. You are in there socialising with them. For me, I have never understood this part, what difference can it make to someone else what is going inside my stomach – beer or water, it makes no difference, I am here chatting and socialising with you, the honest answer is if this is their response, then maybe they are not people you want to be around in your new way of life. They are just not going to fit anymore, you need to be around the people that say, "Water? Yes sure, do you want ice and lemon?"

But as this is the curveball section what if it does go wrong? What if you do have the beer option, which is likely to lead to the kebab or burger option after? The answer is: nothing. The next day you can't change it, you need to move on like mentioned before, and trust me, you will learn from this. The danger is it leads to a second night, then third. It's very common and I have heard it a lot, it's now Saturday night, indoors watching a movie, am I making my omelette, or, since I broke the diet last night, having a take away instead won't hurt will it? After all, I can always start again on Monday. That's where a lot of diets fail - one bad move leads to another. I couldn't even tell you why that is, if you have been on your diet a few weeks and done everything right your willpower is at its strongest, it's easier to say I will make the omelette and not have the take away because you don't want to undo all you hard work, but the minute you fail it leads to more fails. I guess that's just the way we are programmed, so the answer, well, like I said, learn from the mistake, remember the feeling of disappointment the next day and use that as a positive next time.

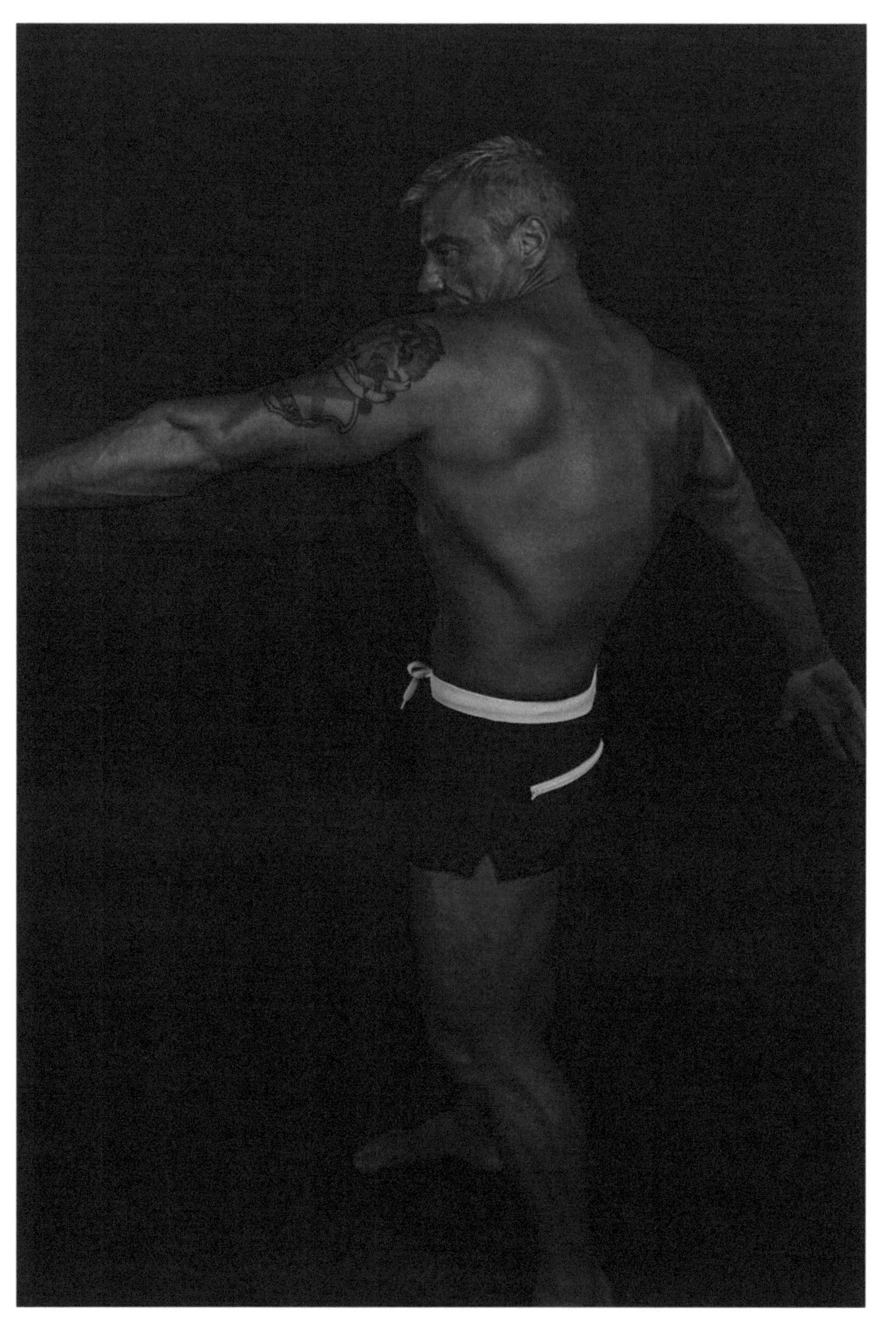

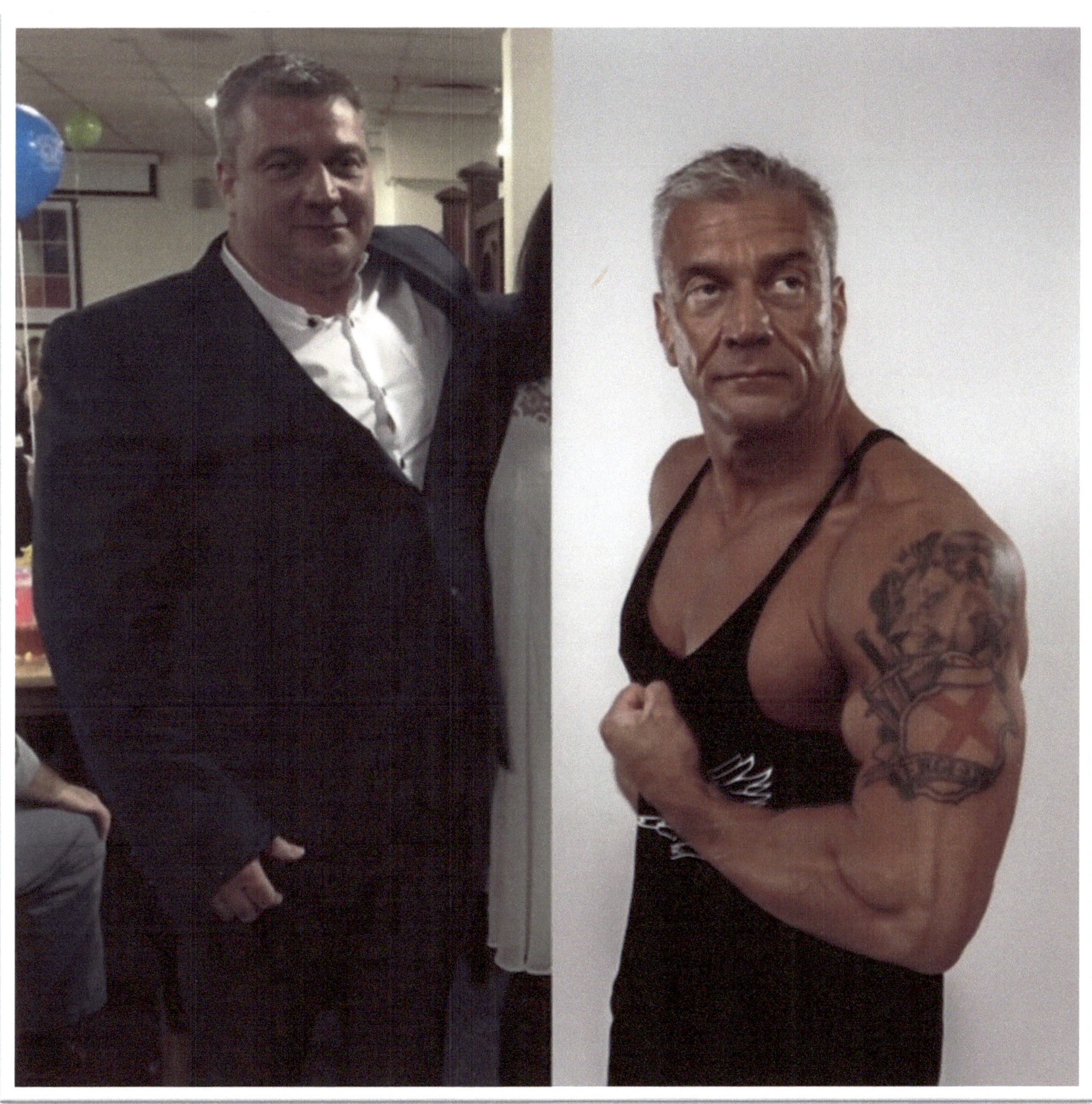

CHAPTER 3: THE TRAINING

The part you have been waiting for, or the part you most bought this book for, right? The training? Well certainly this is the case for me - the gym is the most enjoyable part of my day, that I am sure of.

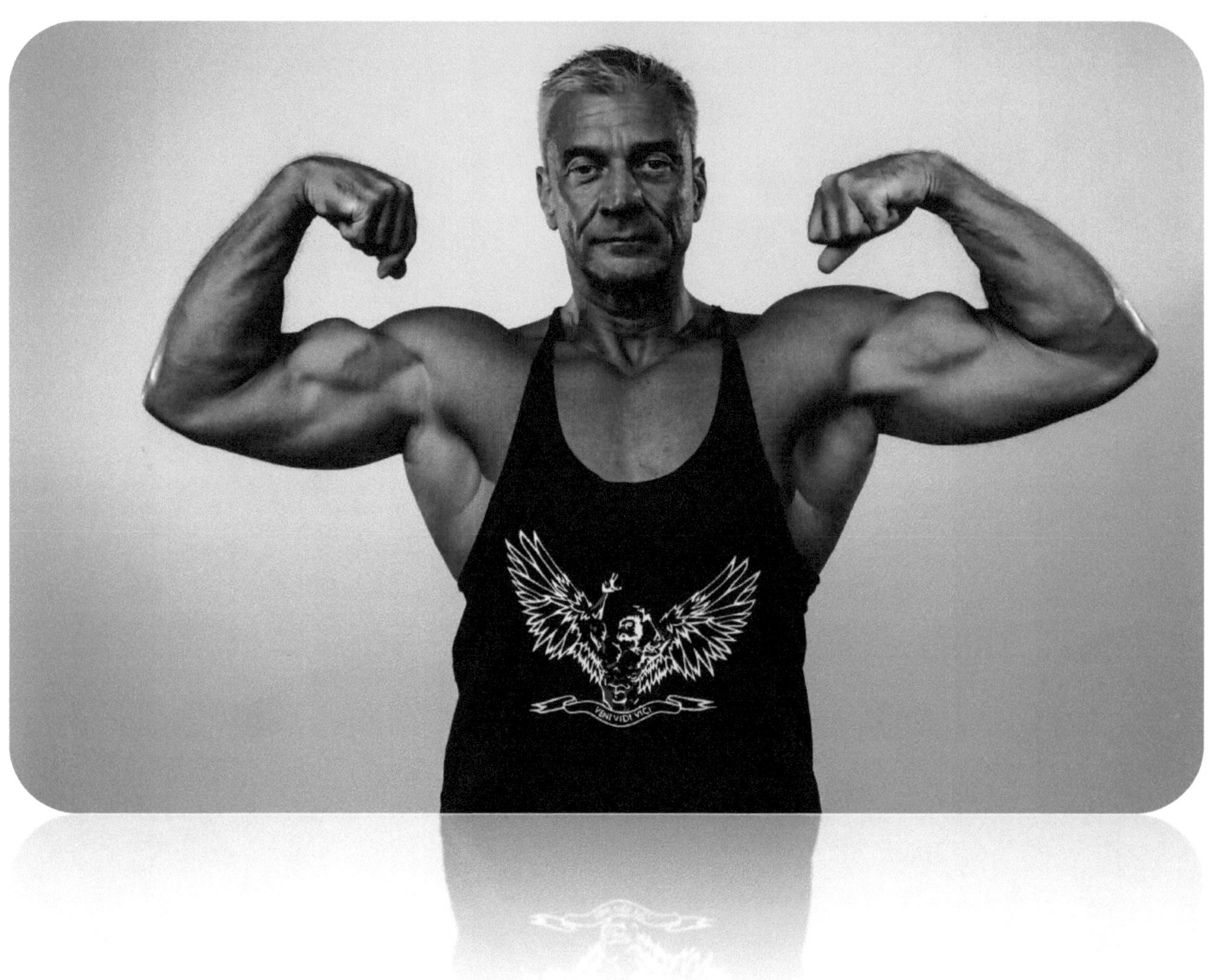

I know I said in the diet section diet was 80% of all this, so without needing a great deal of maths skills that means this part is only 20% which when reading kind of trivialises it.

Obviously this part is much more important than what 20% entails, but, the emphasis is on that fact that you can lose weight with the right diet and without any training but it is not the same the other way around. If you just train, yes, you will gain some muscle, but it won't look great. The training to complete the overall goal is just as important and getting the balance right is important. I have stated this before but I need to be clear: what I don't want to happen to you is you try and follow these routines and because of your lifestyle and schedules you can't maintain this and give up. All I can do is be honest and write down exactly what my routine is and what I do.

The problem is this works for me around my schedule. The good thing is I do a whole range of different things, all taking different amounts of time and needing different things. Like I said, maybe a trip to the gym isn't available to you in the morning so the parts where I do this you will need to swap for something else. The important thing is you stick to the day and times, if you do a run instead of a hit class, great, you have still fulfilled that requirement.

I do different exercises on a 4-week rotation. In this rotation as well as alternating the exercises I alternate reps and time, so where it states 8 to 12 reps heavy, you will do 4 sets of each exercise raising the weight on each set so the 4th set is at your maximum. Care is needed here though; you need to get the right balance of lifting as heavy as you can but maintaining form. A good guide is the last set you should only do 6 to 8 and struggle to complete the last couple without losing form.

You do have an option to do a 5th set which a lot of time I do and make form a little less important than weight. As you have completed your full 4 sets with good form to your maximum weight that is job done but sometimes it is good to add a little more weight and break form to get the sets out, this will help you increase the lifting weight over time for that muscle part. Imagine if your 4th set of dumbbell press for example was at 30kg, for your 5th set raise the weight to 32kg dumbbells, still try and get 8 reps but if form fails after 3 or 4 lifts that is fine, keep doing this every session until you get 8 good reps and to form, this weight can now make up you 4th set and your 5th set goes to 34kg the next time and so on. Swap around which exercises you choose to do for the 5th set and keep it to just 1 or 2 per body part, any more will fatigue you and your other 4 sets with form will suffer if you do more than two 5th sets.

As I have mentioned elsewhere, the Covid 19 pandemic broke out right in the middle of finishing this off and I had to adjust. I won't go into too much detail again but what I did instead was mostly resistance bands and bodyweight exercises (I will do a more detailed section on this in the accompanying videos to give you those tools as I still use the knowledge I acquired to do any home or hotel workouts if I can't make it to the gym), but on release of this book hopefully everything will be back to normal and gyms will be open and running at full capacity. As I wrote that I just crossed all my fingers and toes that it does happen soon. Anyway, what this did give me was an insight into how higher intensity training with less weight as training with resistance bands dictates this way is better for cutting and toning. I did lose some size during this period, but I felt at the end I had never seen my upper torso in such good shape. Once I got back in the gym, I used this knowledge and adapted it for even better results using the free weights and machines alike.

I set the exercises at 45 seconds, you should really have to grit your teeth to complete the last 15 seconds or so but you must complete the full time, getting this right will determine what weight you should be using, fail to complete 60 seconds and it's too heavy, flow past the finish line with ease and it's too light. So, lets train!

Week 1

_Monday

Time	Exercise
05:30am	20min cycle or uphill walk on treadmill and 1-hour yoga class
06:00pm	*Sets 1 and 2 are 12 reps, and sets 3 and 4 are 8 reps.*
Chest	4 sets flat bench barbell press 4 sets incline dumbbell press 4 sets incline flys 4 sets decline press 4 sets cable cross overs

Tuesday

Time	Exercise
05:30am	20min HIIT programme and 30min swimming.
06:00pm	*Sets: 45sec with 60sec rest*
Shoulders	4 sets shoulder press machine 4 sets upright rows (smith machine) 4 sets side raises (dumbbells) 4 sets front raises (long bar on cable crossover) 4 sets rear delts (cable crossover) 4 sets shrugs

Wednesday

Time	Exercise
05:30am	20min cycle or 40min uphill treadmill walk followed by 20min core programme.
Evening	Rest

Thursday

Time	Exercise
05:30am	20min cycle or 40min uphill treadmill walk followed by 20min core programme.
06:00pm	*Sets: 45sec with 60sec rest (unless otherwise stated)*
Arms	**Biceps** • 4 sets seated dumbbell curls • 4 sets standing curls with EZ bar • 4 sets of hammers (dumbbell, alternate arms in same 45sec set) • 4 sets seated concentration curls (dumbbell, 30sec on left arm followed by 30sec on right) **Triceps** • 4 sets on dip machine • 4 sets skull crushers (EZ bar) • 4 sets pushdowns (V bar) • 4 sets push downs (ropes)

Friday

Time	Exercise
05:30am	20min cycle and 1-hour yoga class
06:00pm	*Sets: 8 to 12 reps, heavy*
Legs	5 sets squats 4 sets leg extensions 4 sets leg press 4 sets lying leg curls superset with weighted walking lunges 6 sets calve raises

Saturday

Time	Exercise
Cardio	Rest
11am	*Sets: 8 to 12 reps, heavy*
Back	6 sets of dead lifts 6 sets of T-bar 4 sets seated rows 4 sets pull overs (dumbbells)

Sunday

Rest Day	

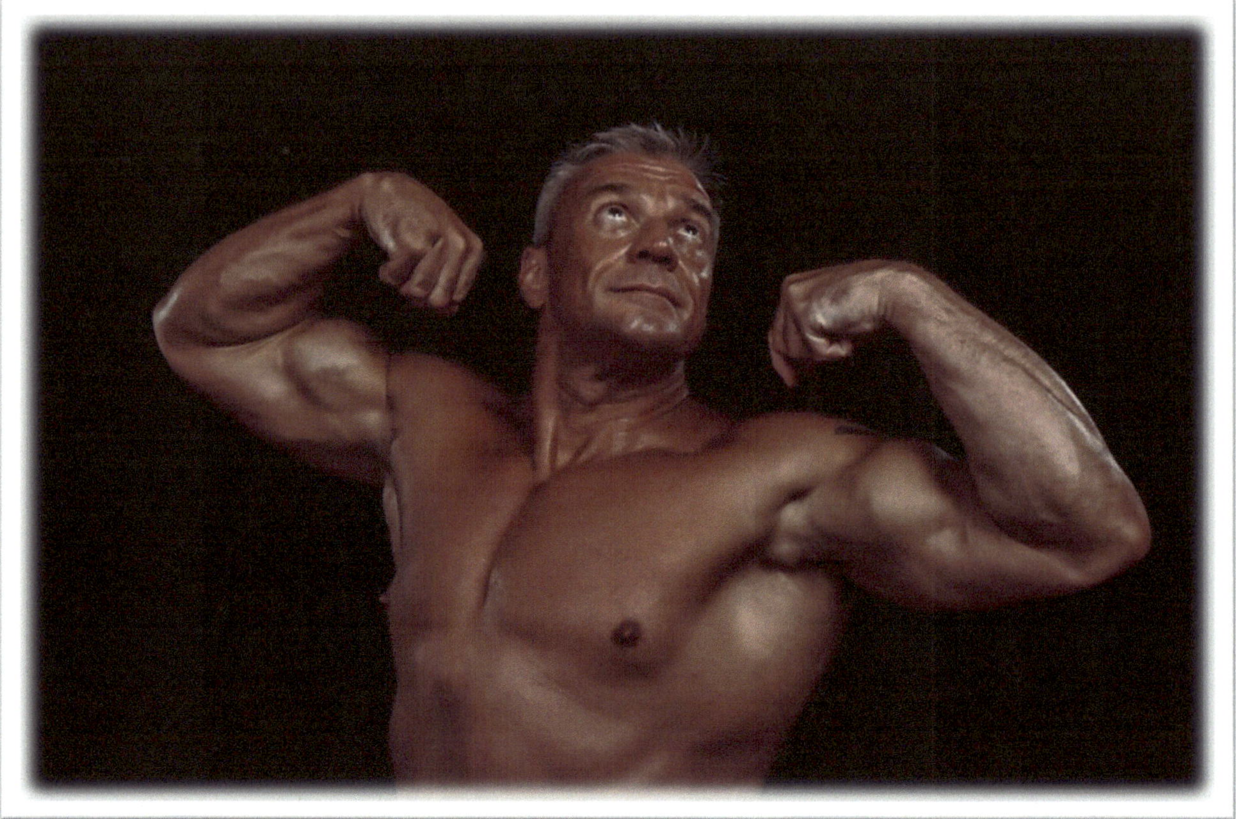

<u>**Week 2**</u>

Monday

Time	Exercise
05:30am	20min cycle and 1-hour yoga class
06:00pm	*Sets: 45sec with 60sec rest*
Chest	4 sets incline chest machine 4 sets incline flyes (dumbbell) 4 sets decline chest machine 4 sets flat press (dumbbells) 4 sets cable cross overs

Tuesday

Time	Exercise
05:30am	20min HIIT programme, 20min core programme and 30min swimming
06:00pm	*Sets: 8 to 12 reps, heavy*

Shoulders	6 sets shoulder press (dumbbell)
	4 sets of supersets with the following 3 exercises one after the other:
	    • front raises (short barbell)
	    • lateral raises (dumbbells)
	    • bent over rear delt flys (dumbbells)
	finish with 4 sets shrugs

Wednesday

Time	Exercise
05:30am	20min cycle, 20min HIIT programme and 20min core programme
Evening	Rest

Thursday

Time	Exercise
05:30am	20min HIIT programme, 20min core programme and 30min swimming.
06:00pm	*Sets: 8 to 12 reps, heavy*

Arms	**Biceps**
	    • 4 sets standing bicep curls (barbell)
	    • 4 sets preacher bar (EZ bar)
	    • 4 sets seated concentrated curls (dumbbell)
	Triceps
	    • 4 sets close grip bench press
	    • 4 sets dips
	    • 4 sets standing extensions (EZ bar)
	    • 4 sets single arm cable extensions

Friday

Time	Exercise
05:30am	20min cycle and 1-hour yoga class
06:00pm	*Sets: 8 to 12 reps, heavy*
Legs	4 sets hack squats 4 sets leg extensions 4 sets leg press 4 sets lying leg curls superset with weighted walking lunges 6 sets calve raises

Saturday

Time	Exercise
Morning	20min cycle, 20 min HIIT programme and 20min core programme.
11am	*Sets: 45sec with 60sec rest*
Back	4 sets of Lat pull downs wide 4 sets seated cable rows (machine) 4 sets bent over rows (barbell) 4 sets pull overs (dumbbell) 4 sets straight arm lat pull downs

Sunday

Rest Day

Week 3

Monday

Time	Exercise
05:30am	20min cycle and 1-hour yoga class
06:00pm	*Sets: 8 to 12 reps, heavy*
Chest	4 sets flat press (dumbbells) 4 sets incline press (barbell) 4 sets incline flys 4 sets decline machine press 4 sets cable cross overs

Tuesday

Time	Exercise
05:30am	20min HIIT programme, 20min core programme and 30min swimming
06:00pm	*Sets: 45sec with 60sec rest*
Shoulders	4 sets shoulder press (dumbbells) 4 sets upright rows (barbell) 4 sets shoulder press fixed machine 4 sets side raises (dumbbells) 4 sets front raises (laydown cable tower) 4 sets kneeling rear delts (cable tower)

Wednesday

Time	Exercise
05:30am	20min cycle, 20min HIIT programme and 20min core programme.
Evening	Rest

Thursday

Time	Exercise
05:30am	20min HIIT programme, 20min core programme and 30min swimming
06:00pm	*Sets: 45sec with 60sec rest*
Arms	**Biceps** • 4 sets preacher bar (machine) • 4 sets bicep curls (EZ bar) • 4 sets side hammers (dumbbells) • 4 sets overhead cable curls (machine) **Triceps** • 4 sets push downs (cable tower with slightly bent bar) • 4 sets kickbacks (dumbbells) • 4 sets overhead rope extensions (cable tower)

Friday

Time	Exercise
05:30am	20min cycle and 1-hour yoga class
06:00pm	*Sets: 8 to 12 reps, heavy*
Legs	5 sets squats 4 sets leg extensions 4 sets leg press 4 sets lying leg curls superset with weighted walking lunges 6 sets calve raises

Saturday

Time	Exercise
Morning	20min cycle, 20min HIIT programme and 20min core programme
11am	*Sets: 8 to 12 reps, heavy*
Back	4 sets weighted back extensions 4 sets of high lat (machine) 4 sets low row (machine) 4 sets close grip pull downs 4 sets Straight arm lat pull downs

Sunday

Rest Day

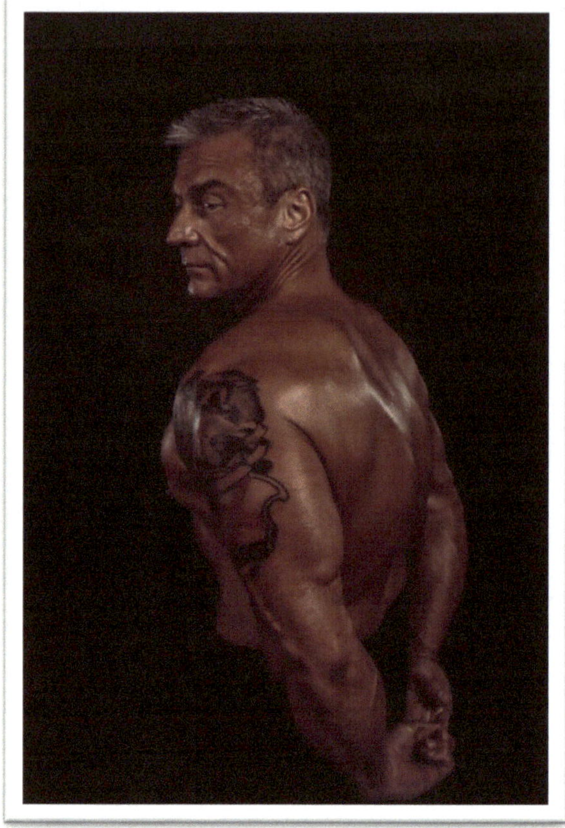

Week 4

Monday

Time	Exercise
05:30am	20 min cycle and 1-hour yoga class
06:00pm	*Sets: 45sec with 60sec rest*
Chest	6 sets incline dumbbell press 4 sets incline flys 6 sets decline press (barbell) 4 sets flat press machine 4 sets cable cross overs (from the lowest position)

Tuesday

Time	Exercise
05:30am	20min HIIT programme, 20min core programme and 30min swimming
06:00pm	*Sets: 8 to 12 reps, heavy*
Shoulders	6 sets shoulder press machine 4 sets upright rows (barbell) 4 sets side raises (cable tower) 4 sets front raises (cable tower) 4 sets rear delts (cable crossover) 4 sets shrugs

Wednesday

Time	Exercise
05:30am	20min cycle, 20min HIIT programme and 20min core programme.
Evening	Rest

Thursday

Time	Exercise
05:30am	20min HIIT programme, 20min core programme and 30min swimming.
06:00pm	*Sets: 8 to 12 reps, heavy*
Arms	**Biceps** • 4 sets seated bicep curls (dumbbells) and superset with standing dumbbell hammers • 4 sets hammers (ropes on cable tower) • 4 sets of 21's (short straight bar) **Triceps** • 4 sets lay down extensions (EZ bar) • 4 sets dip machine • 4 sets push downs)V bar) and superset pull downs (rope on cable tower)

Friday

Time	Exercise
05:30am	20 min cycle and 1-hour yoga class
06:00pm	*Sets: 8 to 12 reps, heavy*
Legs	5 sets squats 4 sets leg extensions 4 sets leg press 4 sets lying leg curls superset with weighted walking lunges 6 sets calve raises

Saturday

Time	Exercise
Morning	20 mins cycle, 20 mins Hitt programme and 20 min core programme.
11am	*Sets: 45sec with 60sec rest*
Back	4 sets of Lat pull downs wide 4 sets close grip seated cable rows 4 sets wide seated cable rows (machine) 4 sets high row (machine) 4 sets straight arm push downs

Sunday

Rest Day

CHAPTER 4: DIET

Or is this part the best bit? Training or diet? I will let you decide. "The fine line," - that's a great saying for this category. There is a very fine line to getting this right or wrong, a very fine line between making the diet too boring and the risk of faltering slithers in, or trying to spice up the diet too much and ending up not getting the maximum results from your training and cardio. I will try and guide you through this minefield as best I can, considering I have no idea your body type, condition or goals but I promise you this is exactly what I did to get these results, not at first (far from it), but hopefully I made all the mistakes so you don't have to, and of course there is also the support programme we offer that you can utilise anytime. So, Let's eat!

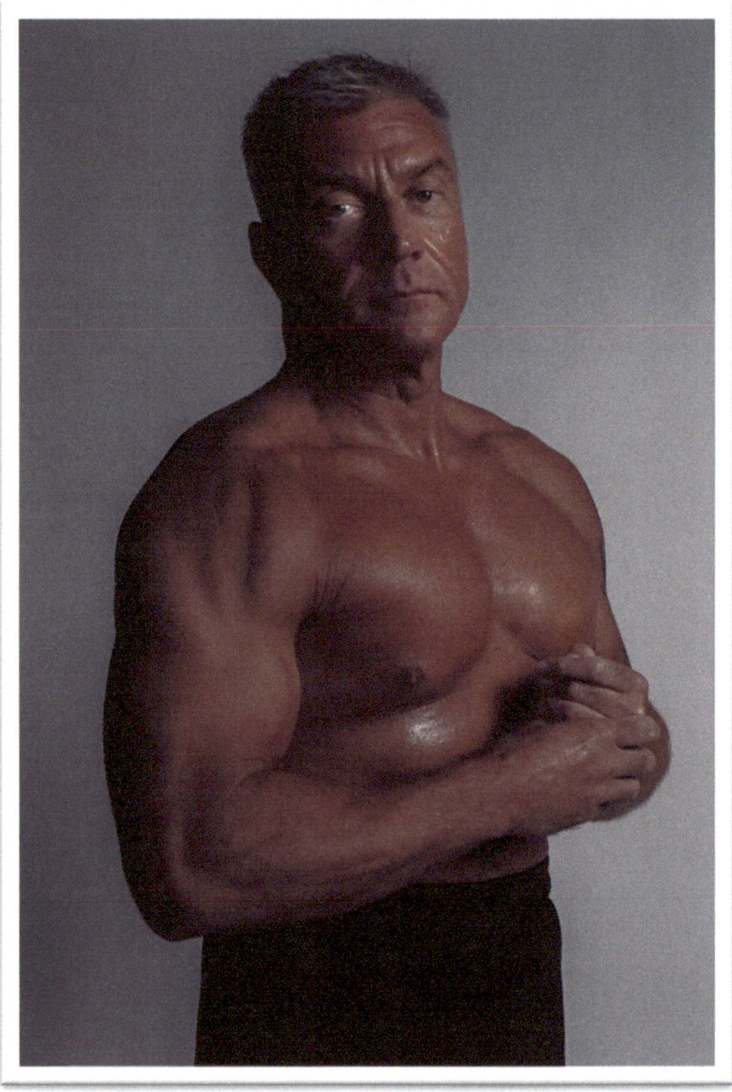

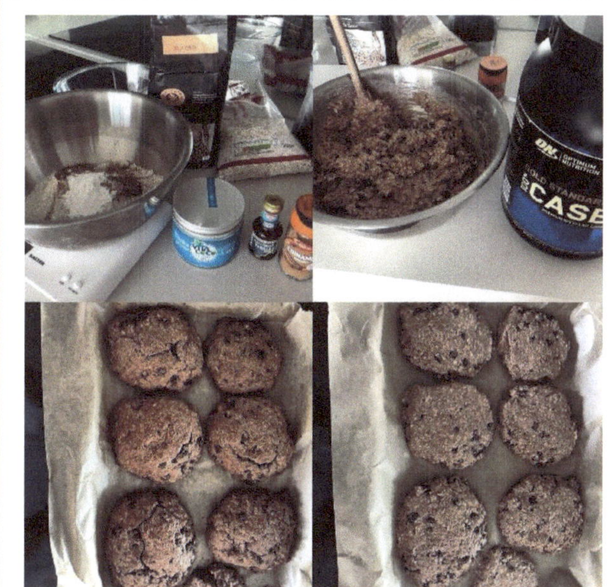

TREATS

If you are going to treat yourself always try and make your own, these protein cookies always satisfy my weekend cravings without sacrificing all of the week's hard work.

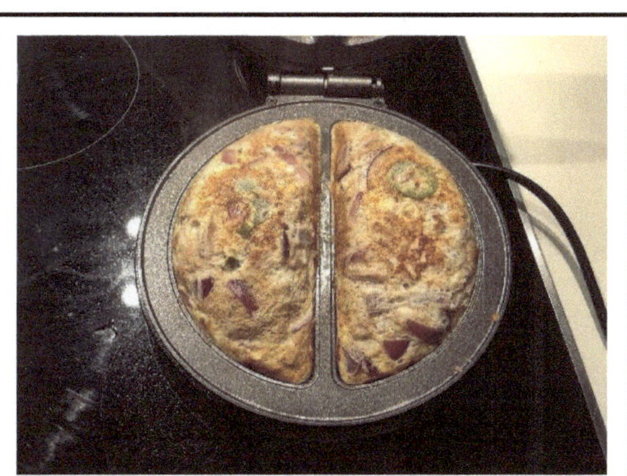

COOKING TOOLS

Invest in the right tools, this omelette maker is perfect for making a very tasty and nutritional meal with easy prep and cleaning

I am sure you have heard it before but I will say it again to emphasise the importance of this, your diet is 80% of reaching your goal, all the cardio and training sessions will be fruitless if the fuel is not correct, and for our age group this is even more so.

If you remember I did have a bit of a rant in the introduction around certain individuals promoting incorrect or rubbish advice to sell a certain product whether that be a supplement or training/diet plans, well, apologies but this section has a rant as well. This one is about certain advice as well: be very careful when planning your diet with certain diet/ fat free products. I think there is more knowledge around these items now than there was when I first started. My advice is don't go anywhere near them - they are a false friend in the worst sense, yes its true they may have 0 calories, 0 fat etc, they can't lie about this as the consumer rights make it law they can't. What they do have to do now is list what they have substituted the sugar or fat with to still give it the taste, but it's not in big bold warning letters like it should be, it is in tiny writing somewhere on the label, and its these substitutes that do the more damage than the original products.

The biggest culprit of this is sucralose, and it is everywhere. I did a lot of research on this as it was in some sauces that was advertised by, yep you guessed it, Mr and Mrs Instagram, saying they can now put sauce on their dry chicken to make it taste wonderful and no longer like diet food, what a revelation right?

Well, there is the confusion – it's advertised and recommended by all these models to make diet food taste so much better, what they don't tell you is it's no good for actually losing weight. Confused? Yes, me too, hence why I researched it and what I found out was, well first let me say I am probably being a bit harsh on the models, what they were saying wasn't actually a lie, they could have this sauce on the meals and not add weight or cause damage because the researchers who tested the product have said it doesn't really show any signs of harming the body as first reported, nor does it make you gain weight, so for them, who already walk around with a six pack its ok as there isn't much evidence of any harm being done.

But here's the thing, what they don't tell you is the very people they are targeting with their marketing, it does have an effect on. They tested overweight people and found if you have a lot of belly fat the reaction of sucralose in your body spikes your insulin and blood sugar levels which then stops your body burning off the fat. I wish I had researched before I bought a selection box of the stuff, half of that box is still in the cupboard!

Maybe now that my journey is complete I may go back to them as they did taste nice, but for you, whilst you are doing your journey and losing the weight keep clear of anything that has these sugar substitutes in them. Then once you have arrived with me at the top of the mountain then you can maybe research and see if it is something you want to add into your maintenance plan, we will discuss it over a green tea on that mountain.

I do want to touch briefly on treats and cheat meals, hopefully without the risk of sounding like a broken record or making you think I am resentful to a certain age group. Those twenty something's I keep mentioning with the high metabolism do have a few get out of jail cards when it comes to their diet, they can have that break or extra cheat and not pay the penalty. Unfortunately, we can't, we will pay for them every time. So, cheat meals and treats, for us, don't really exist, well, not in the form of what first comes into your head when you think cheat meal: pizzas, burgers, Chinese takeout - it's a disaster, you need to accept that to continue, but it's not all bad news so please don't throw this book in the bin just yet. We can and do have cheat meals,

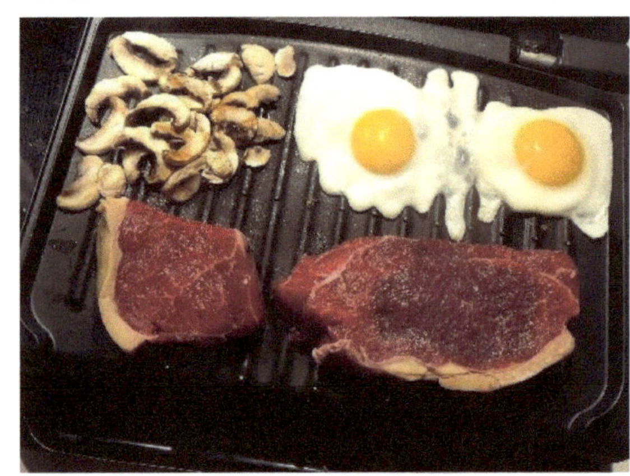

CHEAT MEAL TIME

Don't despair with the healthier cheat meal option than our younger friends. To me this is way better than a pizza or fried chicken, and even when cooking your cheat meal just using the grill which disposes of all the fat helps so much in our weight loss journey.

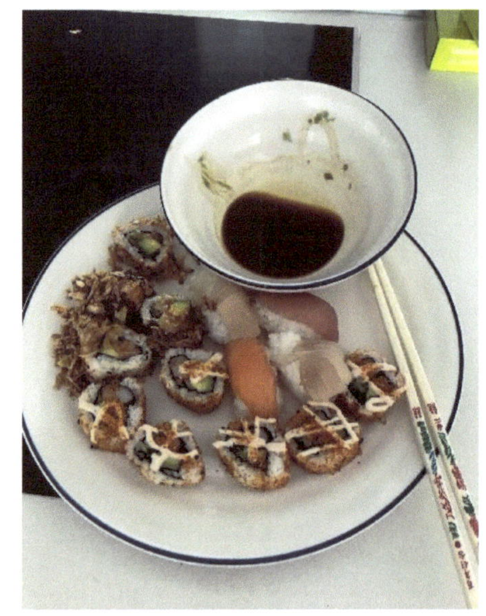

Keep cheat meals healthy without the saturated fats.

just look at them as adult ones, please don't worry - there's steak and potatoes, sushi, pasta and even some bread other than just wholemeal so it's not all bad.

My favourite cheat meal that I usually have on a Saturday night is a large sirloin steak, again purchased from the meat market. Hey, I only get this once a week, I am not putting that in the hands of the local supermarket. I will also cook some boiled new potatoes, garden peas and have some type of bread roll - one of my favourites at the moment is an olive roll or a pecan and cranberry loaf from the deli counter.

Other options available which I have sometimes could be a spaghetti Bolognese, or The Rock's favourite, 'The Sushi Train,' trust me, it's worth checking out his Instagram just to see it!

 Also, by way of treat, every other weekend I will make some protein cookies, I will give you the recipe and instructions for these for you to try them out.

With the exception of the sushi all of these I have are homemade. For me, I prefer this, mainly as if I cook it I know exactly what is going into it, plus as it is my one cheat meal the portion is, well, generous to say the least. But, if you like going out to restaurants then that is ok also, but try to keep to the same basis, a good quality steak restaurant or Italian so you know the food is good quality and well cooked. I know from experience going out and getting a bad meal knowing it's your one treat of the week, that is a low feeling my friend, a very low feeling.

Now let's concentrate on the most important part, the fuel that's going to change your body forever.

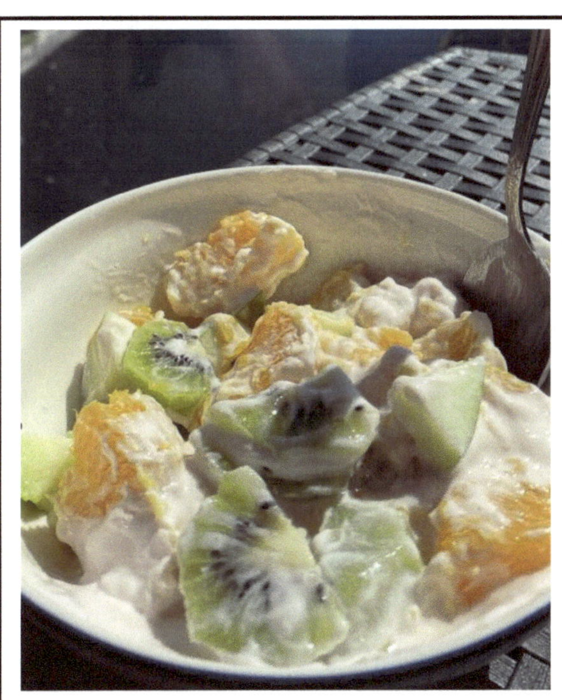

One of my favourites: fruit salad with a 20g protein yoghurt.

I stick with white meat and fish with plenty of vegetables and salad. Like I said before I like to prep the same meals for lunch and put a bit of variety in the last main meal but nevertheless I will still do the plans daily, that way if you feel you do have the time or inclination to make a change you can so. Maybe if it's just one day in the week it won't mess up the rest of the plan.

The salads are pretty much obvious choices: lettuce, cucumber, spring onion and some natural beetroot for colour. There are others so that is your choice and pretty much all salad is great, the other great thing is you can have as much as you want, there is no gluttony where this is concerned although I assume it goes without saying, but salad dressing? NO! I have seen it so many times in the office canteen, "I am being healthy today and having a salad", "Erm, what's all that white stuff all over it?" "Oh, that's salad dressing!' If I was writing this on my phone there would be a whole bunch of face plant emoji's going across my screen. That stuff is riddled with fats, sugar and calories, you may as well go to the chippy for lunch!

With the vegetables for my chicken and salmon I use peppers, red onion, courgettes and aubergine.

For my chicken, before putting it in the steamer I will marinate with turmeric and cumin spice mixed with a freshly squeezed lime. This gives the chicken a real nice colour and acts as a metabolism accelerator.

Now the final part, and the hardest, both for you doing it and for me to give you a timescale or describe as accurately as the past sections. Phase 2 comes into play when you feel the weight loss has slowed down or stopped completely and unfortunately there is no way to give you a time limit which is hard because it is phase, 2 which you need to implement before you reach your goal. Now if your goal is a beach holiday, then you are going to try and judge that as best you can. You may need 4 weeks to finish this off, it may be 8, it really is going to depend on your body type or how well your body reacted to phase 1 and what's left, but bear in mind this part is hard and will take a little longer than you would imagine. A good way to deal with this for the first time, is to track and monitor your results – that means the second and third time you will just get better at it, or maybe you are happy with where phase 1 has bought you and that is perfect, just stay with phase 1.

As always, remember as we get older we will hold extra water and mass so doing phase 2 is only for the beach holiday or a similar goal. The maintenance chapter will cover this a lot better and in a lot more detail as I don't want to overload you at this stage as you are just starting out on your journey.

EXPERIMENT

Never be afraid to experiment. At the end of this section I will give you all the weights, measurements and recipes for everything in this diet but I didn't get these from a book or on the internet, I just experimented, as long as you remember the basics and use the main ingredients of lean meat and fish, with a few exceptions the sky's the limit as far as seasoning and veg is concerned. Just adding some cherry or chopped tomatoes and jalapeños amazes the taste buds!

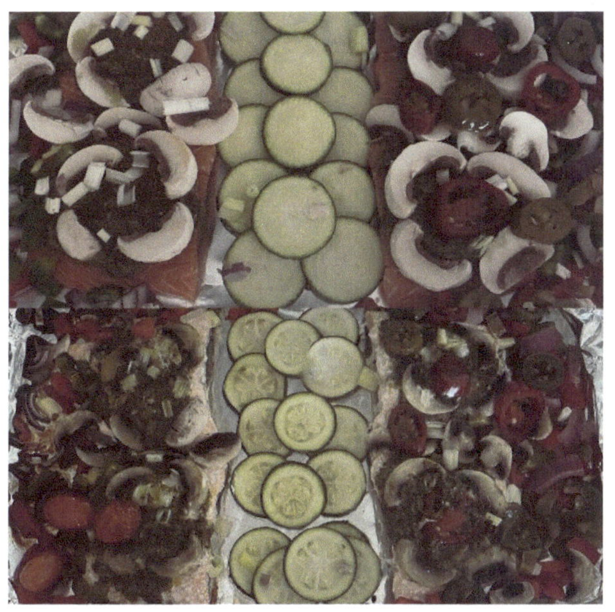

COOKING TOOLS

As with omelette maker if you have the right tools it limits the opportunity to fail, this simple and cheap steamer is a god send for this type of diet, just chop the meat, season and throw in the tray, then the same with whatever veg you want, just chop it and throw in the top section and in 35 mins you have your 3 lunches ready to box up. I also love this item because it's the cleanest way to cook, literally any fat in the meat ends up in the catching tray to throw away making it 100% lean meat that's left.

<u>PHASE 1</u>

Monday to Friday

Fasted cardio Breakfast: (after fasted cardio)	2 whole eggs, 2 egg whites poached and 50g oats made with 2/3 water and 1/3 coconut or almond milk topped with a handful of blueberries, 1 tbsp pumpkin seeds, 2 tbsp chai seeds.
10:30	2 rice cakes with 1 tsp natural peanut butter
1pm	175g steamed chicken or turkey breast, 75g grain or rice, steamed vegetables.
4pm	75g tuna, 2 ryvita protein crackers
6pm training followed by	2 scoops of whey protein
8pm	75g prawns, 25g rice, salad or 100g white fish (my favourite is sea bass) and salad or tuna and jalapeño 3 egg white omelette with salad

Saturday

Fasted cardio Breakfast	Egg white omelette with spinach, red onion and 2 mushrooms, 50g oats made with ¾ water and ¼ coconut or almond milk topped with a handful of blueberries, 1 tbsp pumpkinseeds, 2 tbsp chai seeds.
10:30	whey protein shake 2 scoops, ¼ almond or coconut (unsweetened) ¾ water
1pm	salmon fillets with freshly squeezed lime and Mediterranean veg
4pm	fresh fruit salad with protein yogurt
7pm	cheat meal (See cheat meal in earlier in this chapter)

Sunday

Breakfast	2 slice wholemeal bread, 100g smoked salmon, 2 tbsp black beans, 2 whole eggs
1pm	175g steamed chicken or turkey breast, 75g grain or rice, steamed vegetables
4pm	whey protein drink
7pm	choice of the 3 options from the week selection

PHASE 2

This will be the same for all seven days to strip the final layer off you just before you head to the beach.

Fasted cardio Breakfast	4 egg whites poached, 50g oats made with water, 1 tbsp pumpkin seeds, 2 tbsp chai seeds.
10:30	whey protein shake 2 scoops
1pm	100g steamed chicken, turkey breast or salmon, 25g grain or rice, steamed vegetables
4pm	50g tuna 6pm train followed by 2 scoops of whey protein
8pm	75g white fish (my favourite is sea bass) and salad or broccoli, or a tuna and jalapeño omelette with salad,

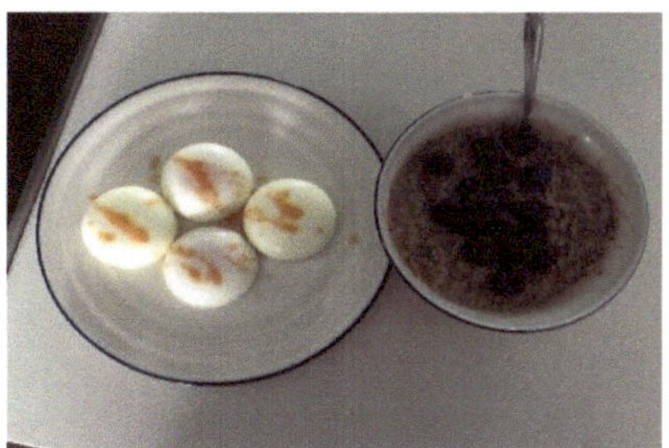

BREAKFAST MADE EASY

For me this is always the best option for breakfast, everything we need on our journey, simple and quick to make.

Protein Cookies

Ingredients:	200g oats
	180g spelt wholemeal flour
	3 tsp baking powder
	3tsp cinnamon
	1/8 tsp pink Himalayan salt
	4 scoops chocolate diet Whey powder
	36g coconut oil
	2 eggs
	2 tsp vanilla extract
	80g raisins
	1/2 pint almond milk
Instructions:	Preheat oven at 190C
	Soak the raisins in a bowl of water
	In a large bowl, mix the oats, flour, cinnamon, salt and protein powder together.
	In a separate bowl, mix the eggs, coconut oil, vanilla and milk together
	Add the mixture along with the raisins into the dry mix and continually beat with a wooden spoon(or you can use a blender, I prefer the spoon as its one hell of an arm workout)
	You may need to gradually add water to bring the mix to a liquid
	Once mixed refrigerate for 30 mins
	Line your baking tray with baking paper and spoon small lumps of your mixture onto the paper and smooth down to a cookie shape with the back of a tablespoon.
	Put in the oven, depending on the thickness and the way you like them (I prefer them well done so they are crispy) they should take around 20 mins.

<u>**Steamed Cumin and Lime Chicken**</u>

Ingredients:	175g diced or cubed chicken
	half of a lime
	1/4 tsp mixed cumin and turmeric
	50g red onion
	40g courgette
	40g red and green peppers
	50g red and white quinoa
	40g black beans
Instructions:	Take the chicken and place into a bowl, marinade with 1/4 tsp turmeric, cumin (you can buy this mixed) and half a freshly squeezed lime, leave this for 30 mins
	While the chicken is marinating prepare the veg cutting into small cubes and slices.
	Once prepared add the chicken to the bottom layer of your steamer and the veg in the top layer and steam together for 40 minutes. Once cooked separately warm the quinoa and black beans and serve together.

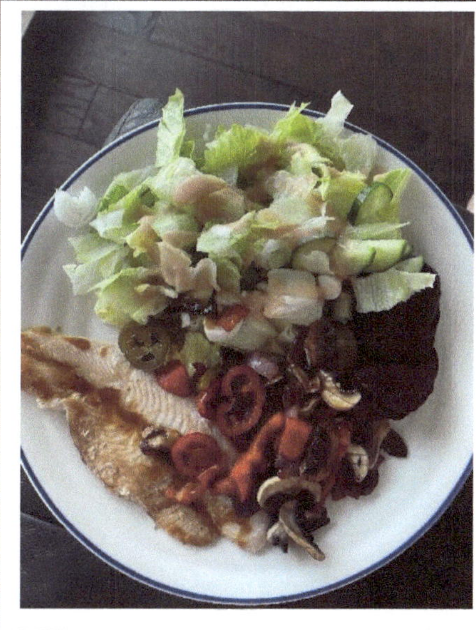

COLOUR

It's amazing how just having vibrant colours in front of you makes the eating part a little less like 'I am on a diet.' As with the lunches experiment with good quality fresh produce making it vibrant and tasty, to liven up the salads my go to garnish is a freshly squeezed lime with a tbsp of balsamic vinegar. Put that with some colour such as beetroot, how nice is that!

Poached Salmon with Pesto and Veg

Ingredients:	1 salmon fillet
	1 tps pesto
	half a lime
	40g mushrooms
	50g green and red peppers
	20g jalapeño
	50g aubergine
	50g red onion
Instructions	Place a sheet of silver lining on a baking tray and place the salmon onto this
	Spread 1 tsp of pesto over the salmon and cover with all the veg
	Squeeze the half a lime over the whole dish
	Cover with silver lining and back in oven for 40 mins.
	Serve with a small portion of new potatoes or brown balsamic rice and garnish with salad.

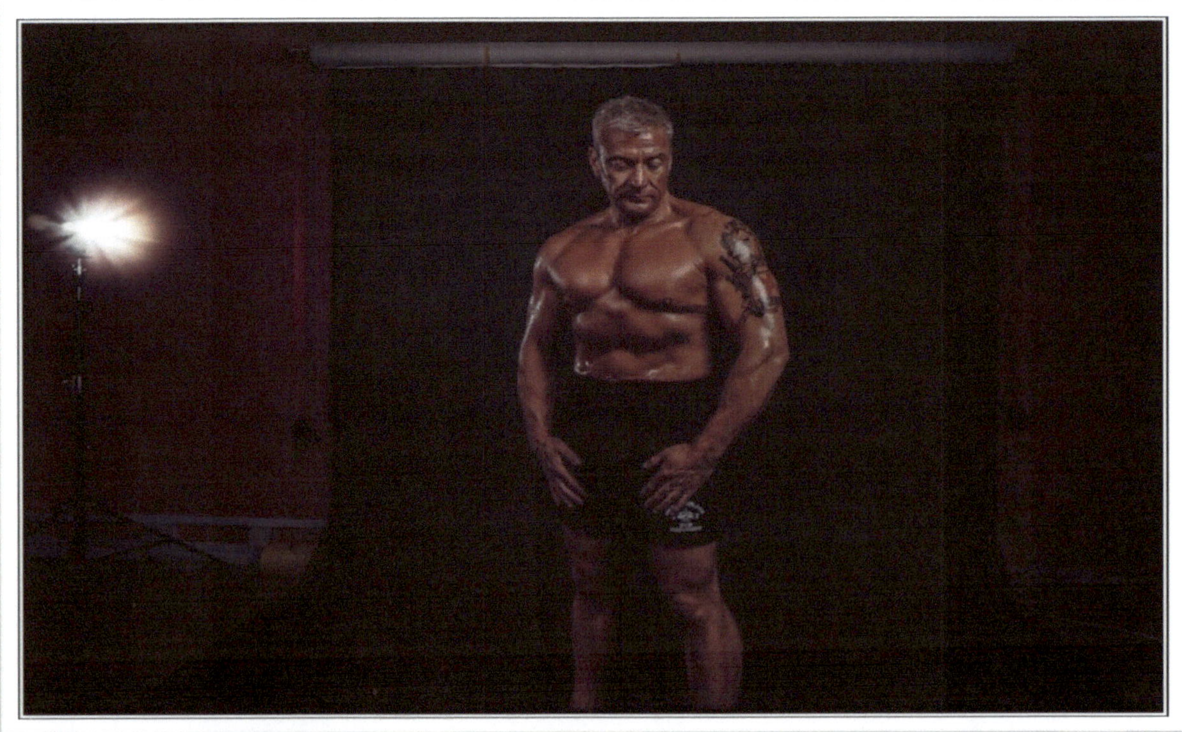

Poached Salmon with Pesto and Veg

CHAPTER 5: MAINTENANCE

Well done, you have completed your journey and you have a new and improved body. I said you couldn't understand the feeling you have right now until you have done it, feels good right? Congratulations, you deserve it, now the less hard part but hard all the same, no falling back into old habits or putting that weight back on because you looked good on the beach once. Remember, this wasn't a diet, this was a lifestyle change, now we can return to life a little more normal, still healthy but with a little less restriction, that's the prize, so here's how we do this. Let's maintain!

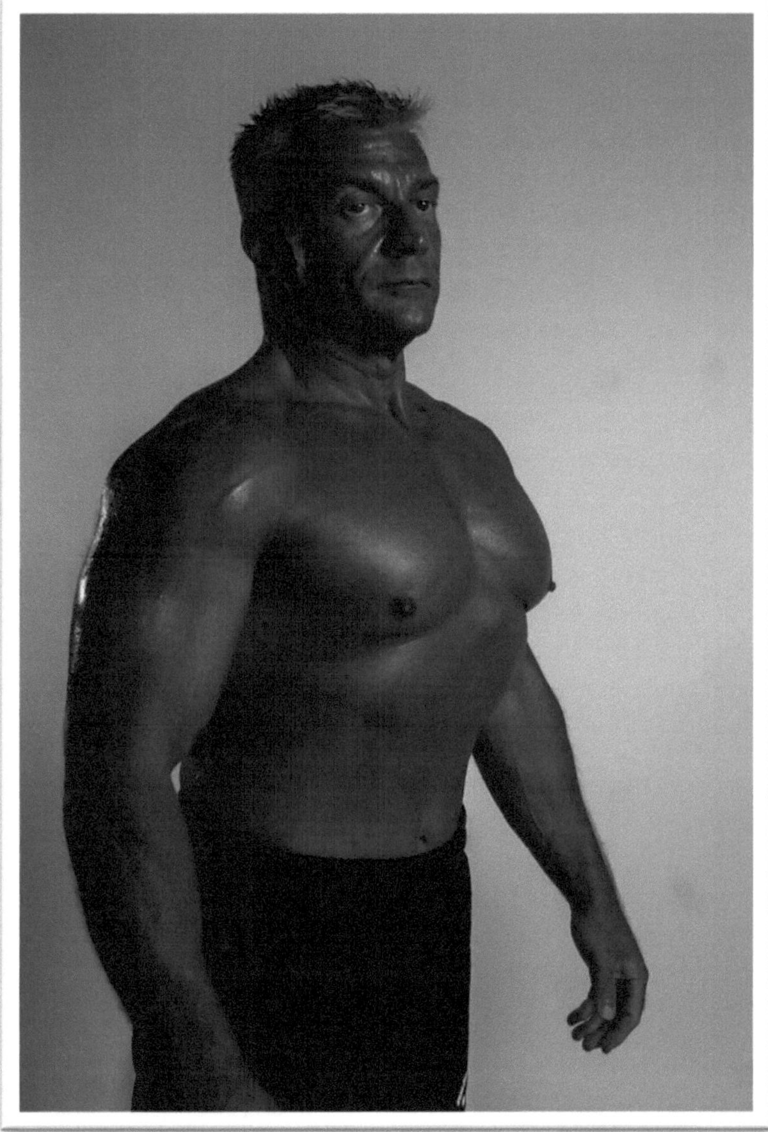

So, you have the amazing body you have dreamed of and worked so hard to get, so congratulations is in order. How do you feel? Pretty amazing, yes. Now let's keep that eh?

This is where this book differs so much to diet plans, because you are going to stay with what you now know and have just learnt, wait, wait, before you throw the book at the wall or look for my Instagram account to hurl abuse (well you can do that, I promise I will give you a dignified answer), let me explain. This part is much more enjoyable, and I can't stress enough if you follow this advice it is so easy to keep all your hard work, that sounds great right? Going from something so hard to something much easier and also it comes with another a massive reward, a cheat DAY! Not a cheat meal, a whole cheat day and still keep the new you that has been parading around the beach, imagine that, a whole day you can literally eat what you want without putting any weight back on or without any guilt.

Let me just point out though, really trying not to be a buzz kill here and burst the bubble I just blew up for you, but please consider the health risk as well. It is ok not putting the weight back on, and you won't with this, but remember, your body is now a temple, to quote the famous phrase – in my mind the last thing you want to do when you have completely cleansed your body is ram it full of sugar and saturated fat once a week as this will just give you other problems. Plus in my experience this can be a slippery slope back to our old ways, if you cast your mind back to when we first started the path to obesity, it didn't happen straight away and all at once, it started with a bad meal here, a junk meal there, so that's why I see that as a danger of going back to that. And to be honest in the new life I don't miss that type of food. I like looking at things like spaghetti Bolognese and pie and mash as the 'bad part' of my diet which is why I have no intention of reintroducing my taste buds to the aforementioned junk.

I will give you an example of the menu on my types of cheat day starting with breakfast: you could have the old fashioned English breakfast, but keep it clean: buy good quality bacon and sausages from the butchers, it is amazing how making a special trip to the butchers for food subconsciously keeps it as a cheat meal, it feels like you're having something special rather than just nipping down the local shop or putting it on your weekly shopping list. Still, grill them all on the fat removing grill, that frying pan still needs to stay in the dark part of your drawers. Also, still poach the eggs but of course its full eggs, all yolk included. Some nice fresh bread and grilled mushrooms. Another treat for breakfast I enjoy is a trip to the local cafe, but not that greasy spoon full of yellow hi-vis (I was a bricklayer so I can say that without any prejudice) and I enjoy salmon and avocado on sour bread with a few extras like black beans.

And for lunch as already mentioned there are so many healthy options: wholesome food, a good quality meat pie with creamy mash potato, a juicy sirloin steak with oven cooked chips, one of my favourite cheat meals is a good homemade spaghetti Bolognese with some slices of garlic bread. The furthest I would go in regards to saturated fat would be on a trip to the seaside, I am definitely having some fresh fish and chips there but that goes in the once in a while treat not the weekly cheat meal. But fried chicken from the man in white, the big M word or pizza, no way is any of that going near me even on a cheat meal/day.

I was quite taken back in the way the government allowed these chains to aggressively advertise their big come back after the Covid 19 lockdown. The adverts portrayed this was the biggest event or the greatest thing to happen, that you could now get this food again, and worse, the fact you can have it delivered to your door again. I really believe this needs looking at and changing as it is a true reflection of where we are going as an obese society and the health risks it is bringing to the future generations, obesity in children is at an alarming figure now and growing, my feeling is as much as we live in a free society and free to make our own choices this part of it needs much more scrutiny and attention from our government.

So, how is this achieved? Well, it really is quite simple, you count your calories for 6 days as you have been doing for 7 to lose the weight and we get that cheat day, you see, now we are maintaining our weight, the correct thing to do is simply eat the same amount of calories as we burn, but as you have learnt with the foods in our fridge and cupboard this will actually be harder to do than you think.

If we go to our base figure of our gym/cardio sessions, we burn 3000 calories. As a test, play with your daily counter and see what you now need to eat of those types of foods to make 3000 calories. Trust me, it will be a lot. So, what I do is I simply maintain 6 days a week on a calorie deficit, now, nowhere near the deficit I had to keep to lose the weight, but, I keep it in deficit all the same. I set mine up at 400 calories under which means for 6 days a week having a 400 deficit. By the time I get to my cheat day which by default is always a Saturday or Sunday which you can swap weekly as it makes no difference which day it is. It is worth mentioning it can be swapped for a week day as well, maybe you have a personal function or work event in the week, remember turning them down, we now you can surprise your colleagues and say YES, I am in!

Anyway, got distracted, where was I? Oh yes, 400 calorie deficit, so, after the 6 days I now have earned myself 2400 calories, add that to my daily 3000 that's 5400 calories I can eat on my cheat day and not gain weight. Now, run to the counter and start punching away and see what a cheat day looks like with 5400 calories at your disposal.

Of course if this isn't for you and you are not fussed about having a cheat day then by all means set your maintenance to the amount you burn each day and just carry on as you have been doing but with something else in the bank, calorie manipulation. This is done by still counting everything as you have done but let's say you get the sudden occurrence, you remember the ones where you had to stay strong, like a friend visiting out of the blue and invites you out to dinner. What? Dinner? But I have had my calories or at least most of them, I can't afford to have a restaurant dinner on top. . . YES you can!

You simply count the calories you had that night and at the end of the day your app will say you are over 550 calories, oh no! Head in hand moment, "What have I done!?" Relax, you are no longer in weight loss mode, this is maintenance mode, this is the easy part remember, all you have to do is ensure you pay back that 550 calories the next day or even the next couple of days if you really went for it, by just cutting something or reducing portion sizes in the next few meals. That's what I do. Say my lunch is 175g of chicken and 75 g rice, well, the next day it becomes say 120g chicken and 50g rice, as long as by the end of the week your calorie intake is where it should be it is all good.

Or another way could be to burn it, now you really need to be with the technology side of the 2 options for this as you could go for a run or do an extra workout to burn those extra calories off which the watch and app will let you know how much work you need to do to burn that treat off. See, I told you this part was easy! Bear in mind though, you still need to maintain that willpower and strength that you have learnt and used to get here. The best advice I can give you is never think you are back to normal, that is the pitfall of diets which is why I keep saying this is not what you are on, yes, you are losing weight but you are losing weight because of your new lifestyle, this is just a natural occurrence of this.

Yes, you will come to a stage where there is no more weight to lose but that is what we call the danger period, when your subconscious starts to tell you I am done, mission complete, and this is where you answer back, NO, I am not done, there is no done, that is the difference between a diet and what you have done and are doing, always keep that in the back of your mind and you will stay this way I promise.

You have earned this, let's keep with it and maintain the ultimate prize, strutting around looking 20 years younger than your age and live the same amount of time longer.

So, that's it, not so hard was it? Don't say or think that for one minute, what you have achieved is nothing short of amazing and you are in an elite category that came back from obesity and an early grave.

 I want to congratulate you with all my heart, you have made it through the book and journey and wish you all the best in the future. Feel free to post your results on this books Instagram and share your results, I will give you a personal shout out and let the world know what we have all achieved together. And lastly thank you so much for buying the book.

There will also be a support mechanism that you can always turn to and use for questions, support or just a friendly come on we got this, we are a family and we will always support each other through the good, bad and hard times, that is what will set us apart from the rest. Lastly there will be videos posted onto our website www.ageisjustanumber50.com with more recipes and training videos in addition to the folder of the 4 week training schedule you downloaded on purchasing this book so ensure you subscribe to the website or our you tube channel @Ageisjustanumber_50.

-- Darren Martin

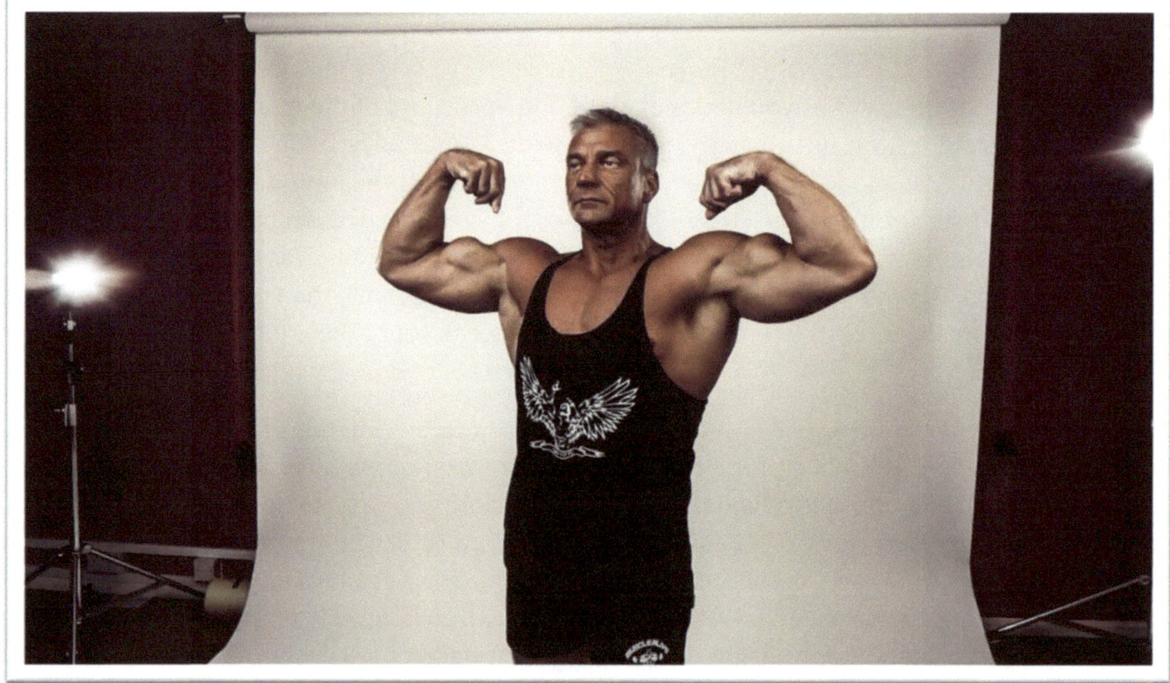

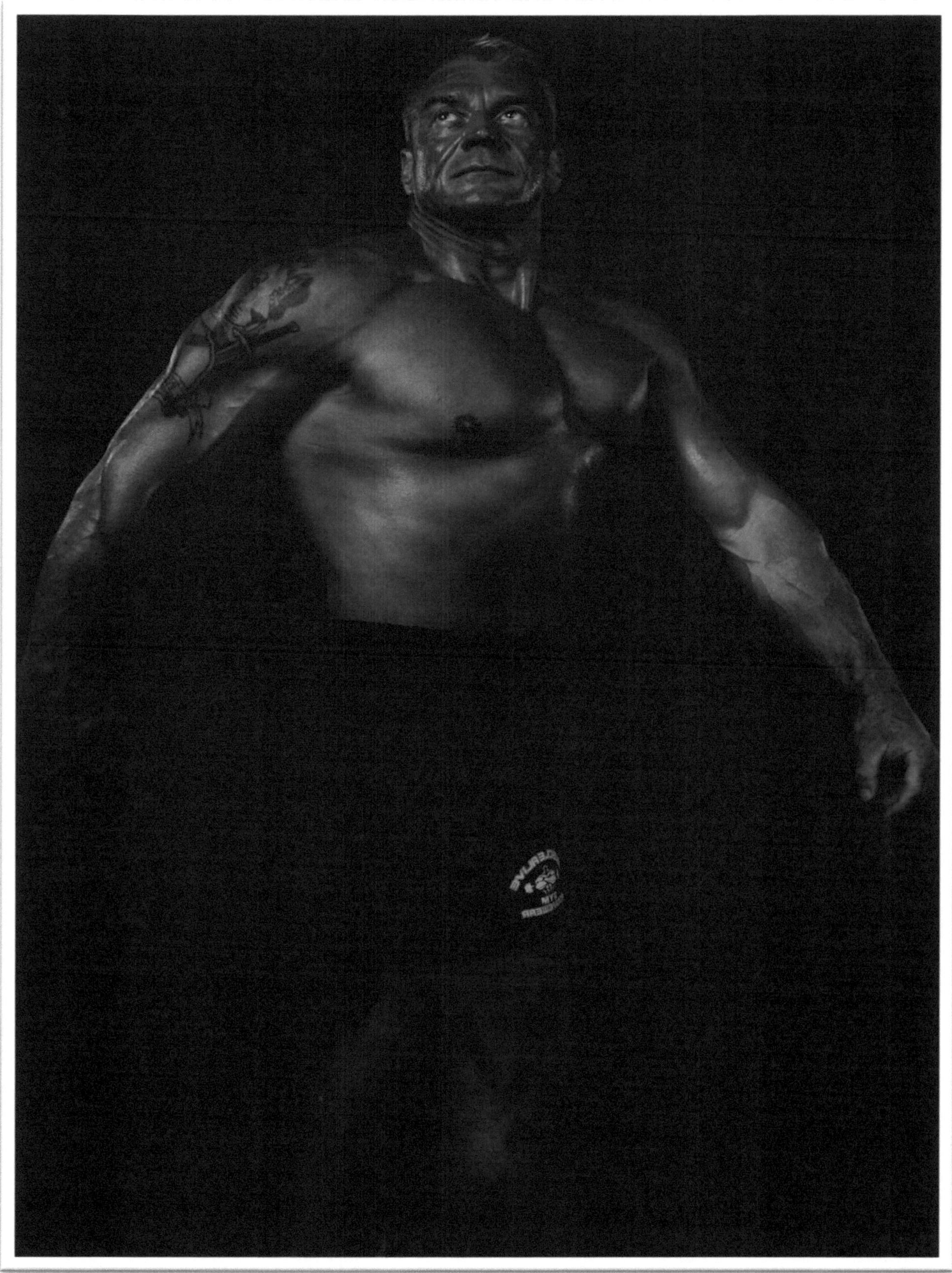

www.ingramcontent.com/pod-product-compliance
Lightning Source LLC
Chambersburg PA
CBHW040143240726
48664CB00002B/577